HEALTHY LIVING
WITH YOUR DOG

21 TIPS FOR A HEALTHY, INJURY-FREE LIFE

DR. BRANDON SCHOMBERG

Live for adventure and stay happy by moving better together.

Copyright © 2025 by Live for Adventure

This book is made with 100 percent human love and dog blessings. All rights reserved. No part of this publication may be reproduced, stored in retrieval systems, or transmitted in any form or by any means, electrical, mechanical, photocopying, recording, or otherwise, or used to train AI LLMs, without the prior written permission of the publisher or a license permitting restricted copying.

Limit of Liability/Disclaimer of Warranty: This book is designed to provide practical information regarding staying active and living healthy with your dog. All the material in this book was confirmed as accurate at the time of publication. It is sold with the understanding that neither the author nor the publisher is engaged in rendering medical advice or other professional services. Consult your medical professional and your dog's veterinarian before starting any fitness and wellness program. While the author has used their best efforts in preparing this book, they make no representations or warranties concerning the accuracy or completeness of the book's content and especially disclaim any implied warranties of merchantability or fitness for a particular purpose. The advice and strategies contained herein may not be suitable for your situation. You should consult a professional when appropriate. Neither the publisher nor the author shall be liable for any loss of profit or other commercial damages, including but not limited to special, incidental, consequential, personal, or other damages. The website links that appear in this book are intended for educational purposes only. The author is not responsible for any information or views on those sites. Please visit www.movebettertogether.com and www.BrandonSchomberg.com for more information on staying healthy and injury-free.

First Edition, June 2025

Published by Live for Adventure

Production Editor: Linda Ruggeri at The Insightful Editor (you championed me, and I'm grateful to get to the finish line)

Copyeditor and proofreader: Jodi Unsinger at Acme Editorial Services (thank you for bringing the words and story to life)

Cover and Interior Design by Miblart

Illustrations by Ellie Glenzinski

ISBN- 979-8-9925454-0-1 (Paperback)

ISBN- 979-8-9925454-1-8 (ebook)

Library of Congress Control Number: 2025906188

To every dog eager at the door—and every human wondering if today's the day. It is! Lace up, leash up, and move together.

TABLE OF CONTENTS

FOREWORD	1
INTRODUCTION	4
CHAPTER 1	9
DOG TAGS: WALKING SAFELY AND STAYING ACTIVE WITH YOUR CANINE COMPANION	
CHAPTER 2	22
THE DOGGIE OATH: A PACT OF LOVE AND LOYALTY	
CHAPTER 3	28
THE LITTER: THE JOURNEY OF RESPONSIBLE DOG OWNERSHIP	
CHAPTER 4	40
HONESTY AND OPPORTUNITY: THE PATH TO HEALTH AND BONDING	
CHAPTER 5	48
PAWS AND FEET: MOVING TOWARD BETTER HEALTH TOGETHER	
CHAPTER 6	59
RUFF AND READY: EXERCISING WITH YOUR PACK FOR A HEALTHIER LIFE	
CHAPTER 7	66
HEALTHY HABITS FOR YOU AND YOUR DOG	

CHAPTER 8 — 76
PAWS AND FITNESS: A DUAL PATH
TO HEALTH AND HAPPINESS

CHAPTER 9 — 84
CORE ESSENTIALS: STRENGTHENING
HEALTH FOR HUMANS AND DOGS

CHAPTER 10 — 96
PROACTIVE HEALTH FOR YOU AND
YOUR DOG: ENJOY ADVENTURES

CHAPTER 11 — 105
ACTIVE LIVES, HAPPY LIVES: INJURY PREVENTION
AND FITNESS FOR KIDS AND DOGS

CHAPTER 12 — 110
HEALTHY AND ACTIVE TOGETHER: EXERCISE
AND INJURY PREVENTION

CHAPTER 13 — 123
HEALTHIER TOGETHER: EMBRACING ACTIVE
LIFESTYLES WITH OUR FURRY FRIENDS

CHAPTER 14 — 130
AGING ACTIVELY: THE SENIOR YEARS

CHAPTER 15 — 150
THE TEMPLE: MOVE WELL, LIVE WELL

CHAPTER 16: 158

CREATING A ROADMAP: EXERCISE ROUTINES FOR YOU AND YOUR DOG

CHAPTER 17 164

HEEL: PROACTIVE PARTNERSHIP

CHAPTER 18 172

TROTTING AND WAGGING: FETCHING IS FUN!

CHAPTER 19 179

WALKING AND OTHER ADVENTURES

CHAPTER 20 183

THINGS TO DO AND OTHER FUN ACTIVITIES

CONCLUSION 188

ACKNOWLEDGMENTS 191

APPENDIX A 192

THE DOG LEASH GUIDE

APPENDIX B 194

THE "PAW"PARED PACKING LIST

APPENDIX C 197

RECOMMENDED WEBSITES

ABOUT THE AUTHOR 202

FOREWORD

We are meant to move. Movement is not just a function of life—it is the foundation of resilience, strength, and vitality. From our earliest steps to the demands of our daily routines, staying active is essential for physical health, mental clarity, and emotional well-being. Yet in today's world, where convenience often replaces effort and sedentary lifestyles dominate, it's easy to forget a simple truth: a body in motion is a body built to thrive.

This book is a powerful reminder of that truth, authored by one of the leaders in our profession, Dr. Brandon Schomberg. Brandon's impact on the field of physical therapy and sports rehabilitation is profound. As a board-certified specialist in orthopedics and sports, a visionary at Twin Cities Orthopedics (TCO), and a passionate advocate for injury prevention, Brandon has dedicated his career to helping others unlock their potential through movement.

What sets Brandon apart is his clinical expertise and the depth of his experiences. Like me, having served in the United States Marine Corps, Brandon's military background has shaped his perspective on health and human performance. In the military, the ability to move well is not optional—it's essential for survival, performance, and resilience in the face of adversity. Both Brandon and I understand the toll that physical and mental demands can take on the body when movement isn't prioritized or optimized. The lessons we've learned from our military service inform every page of this book: the discipline of consistency, the importance of injury prevention, and the necessity of building a body that can endure the rigors of life.

Brandon's work reflects this mindset. Whether leading the TCO Sports Physical Therapy Residency Program, blazing a path as a physical therapist in the military, or mentoring the next generation of therapists, Brandon brings a level of excellence and innovation that has elevated our profession. He understands that healthy living isn't about perfection; it's about embracing sustainable, intentional habits that prioritize movement and resilience. Through this book, he shares practical strategies, grounded in evidence and experience, to help you stay active, avoid injury, and enjoy the freedom that comes with a healthy, pain-free body.

And as Brandon emphasizes, sometimes the best partner on this journey is one with four legs and a wagging tail. Dogs are not only loyal companions but also incredible motivators for movement. Whether it's a daily walk, an energetic game of fetch, or simply being reminded to get outside, dogs inspire us to move and offer emotional support that enhances our overall well-being.

It has been my honor to witness Brandon's journey as a clinician, leader, and fellow veteran. His passion for helping others live healthier lives is matched only by his unwavering commitment to the values instilled through his military service: discipline, accountability, and a relentless drive to improve. This book reflects those values, offering a roadmap to protect your body from injury and discover the joy of movement as a lifelong pursuit.

The journey to a healthier, injury-free life begins with a single step. Sometimes it's taken in formation, sometimes it's alongside a wagging tail—but every step matters. Join Brandon as he leads you through this transformative journey, empowering you to rediscover the strength, resilience, and freedom that come from a body in motion.

George J. Davies, PT, DPT, MEd, SCS, ATC, LAT, CSCS, PES, FAPTA
Professor of Physical Therapy
Athletic Training Department
University of Texas–Rio Grande Valley Edinburg, Texas

INTRODUCTION

This book has been in the making for over fifteen years, inspired by my love for dogs and experiences with dog injuries during my healthcare journey. I have also served two decades in the military and am passionate about fitness. Whether through my clinical practice or my experiences as a soldier, I have always aimed to provide information that helps others lead better lives—this is my *why*. I hope this book contributes to fewer injuries and many memorable moments as you enjoy healthier lives with your family and move better together.

Board certifications, three kids, a wife, several military deployments, and two dogs have led me in lovely directions. The timing for this book feels right today, as mental strength, healthy habits, and physical fitness are crucial worldwide. We can all use more happiness and appreciation for physical freedom. What better way to find it than by spending time with our favorite canine friends? WE LOVE OUR DOGS!

Let's explore ways to stay active with our dogs because that's the goal! Now, let's talk about Dog'ercise. Yes, I made up that word, but let us pronounce it with a thick Southern (or European) accent, emphasizing "Dog" followed by "ercise." Dog'ercise is the key to transforming from sitting home duds to team-fit buds. ROGER that (received and agreed)!

R (Received) O (Order) G (Given) E (Expect) R (Results)

You may notice that I incorporate military lingo and wisdom gained over the years to add motivation and enhance your learning.

Hailing from a small hobby farm in southern Minnesota, I've become a city slicker with a background in physical therapy and experience as a combat veteran. As a self-proclaimed renaissance man, I offer a unique and diverse perspective on life and dogs.

This book is full of goodness and knowledge; use it to have fun while staying healthy, fit, and injury-free for both you and your beloved dog. It's a call to action that combines reflection, laughter, education, and timeless truisms. Exercise is key for our bodies and dogs to stay strong and live healthy lives. So, let's Dog'ercise, remembering the pause in the name. Pay close attention to the 21 Tips throughout the book, which outline the key takeaways.

> Always consult your physician or a qualified healthcare provider before beginning any fitness program, especially if you have existing health conditions, injuries, or concerns.

As you begin, you'll notice the chapters follow a specific rhyme and rhythm. These include:

- Introduction (why this chapter is important for your health)
- Human Element (how the information benefits your healthy lifestyle)
- Dog Care (information that benefits your dog)
- Sample Workouts (with purposeful repetitions here to solidify the routine)
- Educational Insights (those *aha!* moments)
- Story (a tale—pun intended—that you can relate to)

- Recommendations and recommended items (implementation cues)
- Summary of living healthy with your dog

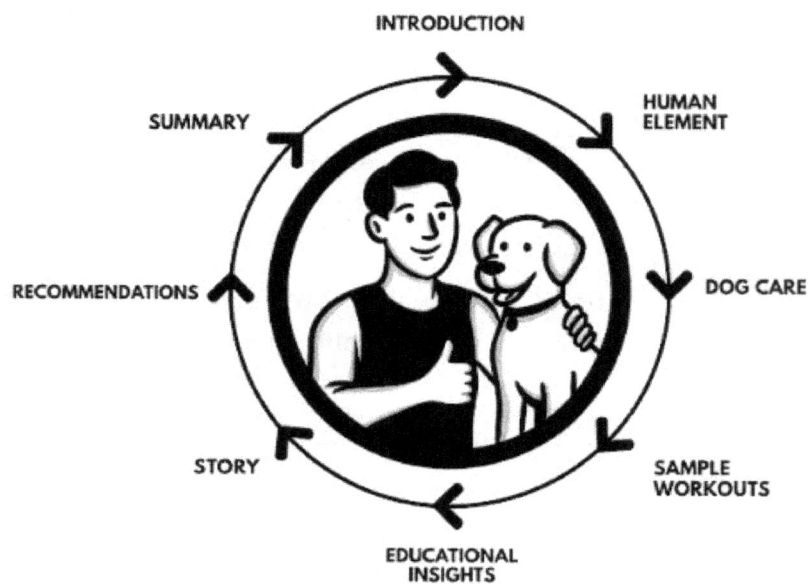

The sequence of chapter sections in this book

In summary, this book is a guide to having fun, getting active, and exercising with your dog by moving better together. With educational insights, starting points, life lessons, and ideas, let's take it Oscar Mike—on the move! Together, we can share these tips among fellow tribes and dog packs and see how quickly goodness spreads among us dog lovers. Not everything will apply to you, so use what makes sense and feel free to discard the rest. Most importantly, enjoy and learn!

If you don't prioritize time for moving better together, you may be forced to find time for disease and sickness later in life.

—Dr. Brandon Schomberg

21 TIPS FOR A HEALTHY, INJURY-FREE LIFE

TIP #1: Stay alert. Stay safe.

TIP #2: Never make excuses. Embrace failures.

TIP #3: Be honest. Seek opportunities.

TIP #4: Execute an action plan. Visualize success.

TIP #5: Support your pack. Increase goodness.

TIP #6: Match activity levels. Establish resets.

TIP #7: Know your age. Stay injury-free.

TIP #8: Build a strong core. Fortify your foundation.

TIP #9: Be proactive. Stay tuned up.

TIP #10: Active lives are happy lives. Have Fun!

TIP #11: Movement is medicine. Build your team.

TIP #12: Progress slowly. Results are achieved.

TIP #13: Prioritize time. It's a lifestyle.

TIP #14: Be the captain. Create inertia.

TIP #15: Drive on. Do not rust.

TIP #16: Move. Maintain inertia.

TIP #17: Know thy body. Marvel and appreciate.

TIP #18: Create a roadmap. Establish a routine.

TIP #19: Be wise. Proceed safely.

TIP #20: Innovate. Be intentional and present.

TIP #21: Maintain companionship. Seek adventures.

CHAPTER 1

DOG TAGS: WALKING SAFELY AND STAYING ACTIVE WITH YOUR CANINE COMPANION

Dogs bring joy. Sustaining an injury while with your dog can be frustrating. Injuries can be costly, resulting in lost wages, expensive surgeries, or the loss of freedom during recovery. This can disrupt your happiness and limit your social life and time with friends and family.

This book aims to promote self-awareness and provide you with practical tips for a healthier life, helping you avoid injuries. Happiness is key for yourself and your dog, plain and simple. You may find this surprising, but this is a familiar scenario for medical professionals. As I have said repeatedly to many of my patients over many years, *"The number one cause of injuries among older adults is while outside walking their dogs."*

What!? Did you say walking outside with your dog is the most common cause of injuries in older adults? I sure did. This is the premise of the foundation for this book. It's written from the perspective of a doctor of physical therapy, a combat army veteran, a model citizen (OK, I made that part up), and someone who just loves being outside with his family and dogs. This chapter focuses on educational content, while later chapters include sections on humans, dogs, and workouts featuring examples and stories that illustrate the benefits of a healthy lifestyle.

HUMAN ELEMENT

Walking your dog should be a simple and enjoyable activity. However, a 2019 publication in the *Journal of the American Medical Association* indicates that the incidence of fractures among older adults has more than doubled since the early 2000s due to injuries sustained while walking dogs.[1] This resonates deeply with me, as I have witnessed and helped rehabilitate numerous senior patients who suffered injuries while walking dogs. Our health is paramount, and preventing injuries while maintaining an active lifestyle is crucial. This means being mindful of the risks and learning proper safety techniques.

Did you know that well-documented research demonstrates a direct relationship between muscle strength and physical activity? This relationship can result in a lower risk of dying prematurely by 10–20 percent. Consistent physical activity can not only prevent muscle weakness but also *reverse* weakness and build muscle proteins—as we say, "put the meat on the bone," to improve your strength and ability to tackle life's challenges! Just ask anyone who has experienced an injury, prolonged illness, or surgery. The result is improved functional movement, allowing you to stay attuned to life's adventures.

---

[1] Pirruccio, K., Yoon, Y. M., and Ahn, J. "Fractures in Elderly Americans Associated With Walking Leashed Dogs" *JAMA Surgery* 154, no. 5 (2019): 458-459.

CAUTION: If you use a cane or walker while walking your dog, I strongly advise you to ensure you can maintain proper control and balance. Additionally, your dog should be well-behaved, especially if you're recovering from an injury or have a balance-assisting device.

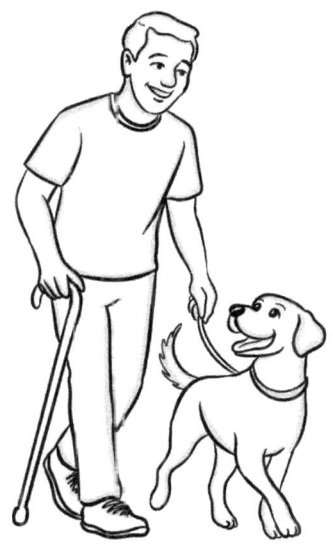

Take all necessary precautions if you use a cane or walker when walking your dog.

DOG CARE

Our dogs require purpose, attention, and lots of love. They're our family, and we all strive to meet their needs. Exercise is also crucial for dogs, as it helps keep them healthy, happy, and well-behaved. Experts generally recommend 30 minutes–2 hours of physical activity a day for your dog, depending on their breed and age.

Research indicates that dog owners walk an average of 22 minutes longer each day than those without dogs, resulting in over 2,700 additional steps at a moderate intensity.[2] According to the American College of Cardiology Foundation (ACC) and the American Heart Association (AHA), this benefits the dogs and significantly reduces the owner's risk of heart conditions.

However, when exercising with dogs, it's important to be aware of potential injuries. Common issues include ligament sprains, muscle strains, fractures, and dislocations. These injuries often result from distractions, uneven terrain, or sudden movements made by the dog. By remaining vigilant and using proper techniques, you can ensure a safe and enjoyable exercise routine for you and your canine companion.

SAMPLE WORKOUTS

> CAUTION: Always consult your physician or a qualified healthcare provider before beginning any fitness program, especially if you have existing health conditions, injuries, or concerns.

This is a simple yet effective workout routine for you and your dog as you begin. This workout requires about 35 minutes:

---

[2] Dall, P. M., Ellis, S. L. H., Ellis, B. M., et al. "The Influence of Dog Ownership on Objective Measures of Free-Living Physical Activity and Sedentary Behaviour in Community-Dwelling Older Adults: A Longitudinal Case-Controlled Study." *BMC Public Health* 17 (2017): 496.

1. Warm-Up: Start with a brisk, 5-minute walk to get your blood flowing. This gets the muscles ready for more intense activity.
2. Interval Training: Jog for 2 minutes and then walk for 1 minute for a total of 20 minutes. This maintains an elevated heart rate and burns calories.
3. Strength Training: Locate a safe space to perform bodyweight exercises. Let your dog rest or play nearby. Do 2–3 sets of the following exercises:

   - 15 squats
   - 10 push-ups
   - 20-second plank

4. Cooldown: Finish with a 5-minute walk, followed by gentle stretching for you and your dog.

EDUCATIONAL INSIGHTS

Consistent and proper training can help reduce injuries. I have seen, heard, and assisted in rehabilitating many patients who sustained injuries while walking their dogs. The focus is on resolving this dog-walking dilemma and keeping you injury-free. So pack your rucksack because we're going on a journey to maintain our freedom, my DOG LOVERS!

In my military background, I always had a battle buddy, my confidant and comrade for missions. I have always considered my dog as my battle buddy and my dogs as my troops. They are our comrades in our shared endeavors.

First, let's attack your health. This is the most crucial battle I want you to prepare for. Flight attendants remind you to secure *your* oxygen mask before assisting others. In other words, help yourself so you can more effectively help others

What is Exercise? Movement. Let's first grasp this concept.

Remember that as a dog owner, you walk 22 more minutes a day than the average person. That's great! Many of you do even more, but this is excellent news for those considering a canine companion.

Walking for 22 minutes daily has been correlated with more than 2,700 additional daily steps at a moderate intensity—a brisk walking speed. According to the ACC and AHA, owning a dog is associated with a decreased risk of heart conditions[3]—that's amazing! This sounds like a great way to improve your health, heart, and mind.

Injury Alert: Stay alert and keep your knees slightly bent, maintaining a "soft knees" position. This helps protect your knees and enhances body stability, reducing the risk of falls. Collisions between humans and dogs occur frequently in dog parks; keeping a slight bend in your knees will help protect them from injury during a collision, making you steadier on your feet.

---

[3] Levine, G. N., Allen, K., Braun, L. T., Christian, H. E., Friedmann, E., Taubert, K. A., Thomas, S. A., Wells, D. L., and Lange, R. A. "Pet Ownership and Cardiovascular Risk: A Scientific Statement From the American Heart Association." *Circulation* 127, no. 23 (2013): 2353-2363.

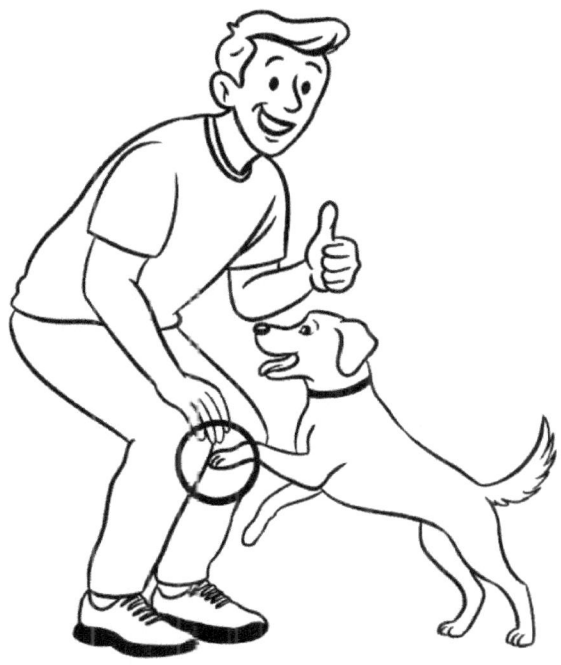

For your safety, maintain a "soft knees" position

Returning to the story of walking with our dogs, considering the numerous injuries I have witnessed over the years, the statement, *The number one cause of injuries among older adults is while outside walking their dogs,* couldn't be more accurate. "Well, what types of human injuries can occur from walking a dog?" you ask. Here's a partial list:

- Various ligament sprains and muscle strains throughout the body
- Quadriceps (large thigh muscle) ruptures and carpal bone (wrist) fractures, often caused by tripping hazards, such as leashes or obstacles

- Patella (knee bone) dislocations or fractures from direct falls on the ankle, shoulder, and wrist
- Lower back and disk herniations
- Collisions at parks—where your dog thinks you're blocking the end zone, there are only a few seconds left in the game, and there is no stopping them from running through you
- Falls occurring due to inattention to uneven terrain, obstacles like raised curbs, tree roots, or hazardous environmental conditions such as ice, resulting in bruises and cuts.Ouchy!
- Leash injuries such as rope burns, falls, or dislocated elbows or shoulders from excessive pulling or force. That rabbit or squirrel teased them just enough!
- Broken pelvis or hips, particularly in older adults
- Head injuries from a faceplant or whiplash

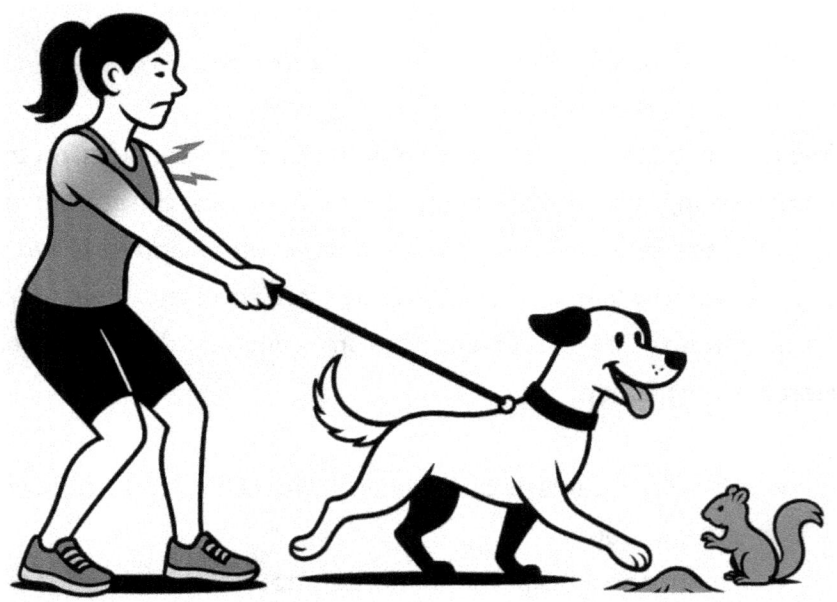

Let's avoid this!

> Fractures are broken bones, and many people use the terms *fracture* and *broken bone* interchangeably. *Fracture* is a medical term. Patients have said, "I don't have a broken bone—I have a fracture," or vice versa. Now you know!

As you can see from the above, we've seen it all in orthopedics and medicine; most of the time, we're simply trying to keep our dogs active. Unfortunately, it's often that we humans end up getting hurt. On the other hand, most dogs are quite agile and less prone to injuries. There's no need to hide in a bubble, though; you just need to follow the tips in this book to reduce your risk of injuries.

Many of these accidents sound terrible and chaotic. That is what we call in the military—listen up, folks—a MUBAR, which stands for "messed up beyond all recognition," substituted from FUBAR, of course. Use your imagination on the R-rated version. Some of you may be in disbelief: "Why would I ever get a dog? Those injuries sound awful!"

Many dog owners simply need to improve their situational awareness of their surroundings. To enhance your safety, it's important to address basic behaviors like distractions and a lack of environmental awareness. In the military, we must be keenly aware of our surroundings so that we return alive from the battlefield. *Stay awake, stay alive*, was our common adage in basic combat training.

"Seems like common sense," you say. "I'll just look around more as I walk." That's a great start, so please keep it up to help prevent injuries. The more vigilant and alert you remain, the better you'll understand the various elements of your current situation, including your perception and comprehension of elements that could lead to unforeseen events or injuries. At times, you may need to approach your environment with caution— or even stop altogether—to prevent injury. This will shift focused awareness of your situation, allowing you to gather information, remain observant, and stay attuned to all details within the environment. This way, you can quickly react to avoid injury. Keep your head on a swivel, my friends.

TIP #1
STAY ALERT. STAY SAFE.

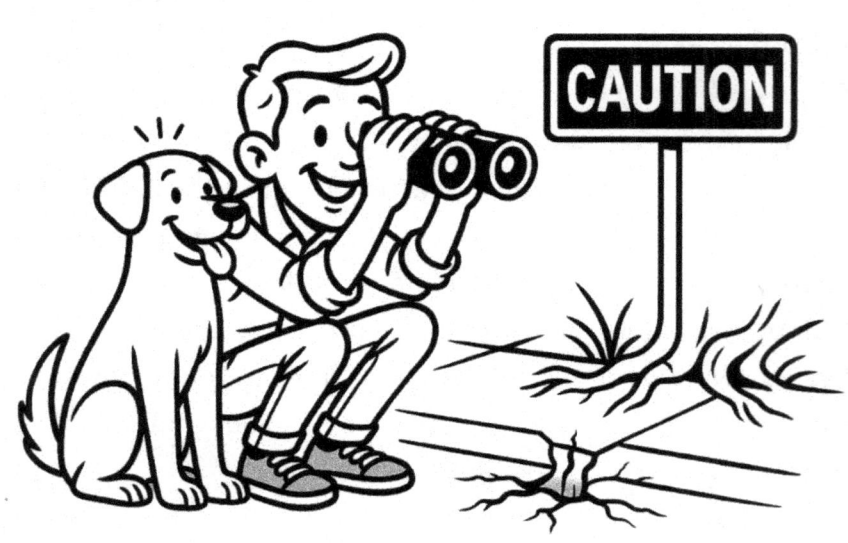

Always remain vigilant and alert in your environment

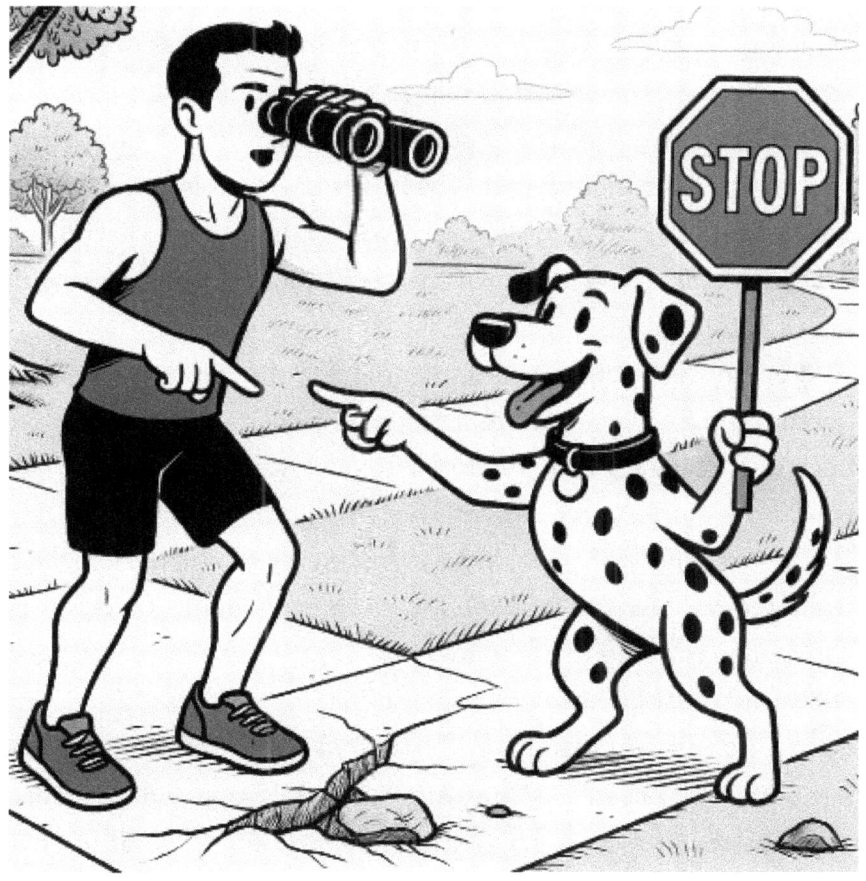

Approach your surroundings with caution. Watch your step!

STORY

Linda, a resolute dog owner, was walking her energetic Labrador retriever, Max, when she tripped over an uneven sidewalk and sprained her ankle. Determined not to let this happen again, she started observing her surroundings more closely. She now enjoys her walks with Max more than ever since she's injury-free.

Imagine you're walking your dog in the park, lost in thought and unaware of your surroundings. Suddenly, your dog spots a squirrel and takes off. The abrupt pull catches you off guard, and you stumble, spraining your wrist. This scenario is common but preventable. By staying aware of your surroundings and using a secure leash, you can prevent such injuries and enjoy your walks safely.

For some people, this concept may be difficult to fully understand and incorporate into their lives, as it may not have been part of their training or upbringing. However, this awareness can be developed over time. Before you jump to conclusions and stop interacting with your dogs, you must weigh the risks against the rewards. The tips provided in chapter 2 should be our *core* values (I was going to name them Dr. Dog Rules but took a more subtle approach). These tips are essential for living a healthier life. Following these guidelines will help you maximize your physical freedom. The essence of these guidelines is that we play safe, stay healthy, stay moving, live for adventure, and what we like to call Dog'ercise fun.

RECOMMENDATIONS

- Stay Vigilant: Always stay alert of your surroundings while walking your dog.
- Use Proper Equipment: Invest in a sturdy leash and harness to maintain better control of your dog. For more information on the best-fitting leashes, check out the website www.movebettertogether.com for details and Appendix A for a summarized version.

- Strengthen Your Body: Exercise regularly to improve your strength and balance.
- Educate Yourself: Learn about common injuries and how to prevent them.
- Consistency: Incorporate regular walking and exercising with your dog into your daily routine.

SUMMARY

Staying active with your dog is a rewarding experience that benefits both of you. However, it's essential to be mindful of potential risks and take measures to prevent injuries. By staying vigilant, using appropriate gear, and following a regular exercise routine, you can have many safe and enjoyable adventures with your furry friend. Remember to "stay awake, stay alive," and keep moving forward, one tail wag and paw salute at a time.

CHAPTER 2

THE DOGGIE OATH: A PACT OF LOVE AND LOYALTY

The love, laughter, and joy that a dog brings into our lives are immeasurable. These loyal companions enrich our days with their playful antics, unwavering devotion, and unique personalities. As we welcome a dog into our family, we must acknowledge the responsibilities that come with this decision. As we commit to caring for our dogs, they, in turn, pledge to be our faithful friends and protectors. This chapter highlights the mutual promises that establish a happy, healthy, and fulfilling relationship between dogs and their human families. Please refer to Appendix C for reputable websites to assist your research and family decision in choosing the right dog. Dog ownership is a huge responsibility!

HUMAN ELEMENT

DOG FAMILY OATH

As dog owners, we must take a "Doggie Oath," pledging to ensure the well-being of our furry friends. This commitment includes providing a safe environment, ensuring regular veterinary care, and dedicating time for training and play. By offering daily love and affection, we support our dog's overall health and happiness. Responsible dog ownership also means being considerate of others by managing our dogs' behavior and keeping public spaces clean. Our dedication to providing our dogs a loving and nurturing home is rewarded with their steadfast loyalty and joy.

DOG CARE

DOG OATH

Dogs, in their own way, take an oath of their own. They promise to be loyal, playful, and always ready to accompany you, offering protection and endless fun. They instinctively guard their families and homes, providing security through their barks and presence. Dogs also play a crucial role in encouraging physical activity, as their boundless energy motivates us to remain active. They pledge to be our best friends, offering unconditional love and companionship, making each day brighter and more enjoyable.

Tail A'la Wishing "Promise" Oath

I promise not to pee inside the house. I promise not to toss flatulence bombs or to fart constantly while sitting on your lap or next to you (this happens all the time). I promise my farts will not stink like a garbage pit or a dead squirrel (eww).

> If a patient passes gas during treatment, I like to lighten the mood by asking, "Was that you or me?" This usually breaks the ice. I'll say the same thing to my dogs, but they usually don't answer me.

I promise not to roll around in snake skins, poo, fish guts, and the list goes on (yes, that happens—what?!). I promise not to start a kitchen fire and knock over the garbage. I promise not to jump on every houseguest or anyone else, for that matter. I promise not to chase the neighbors, kids, or mail carrier. Really, I will try.

I promise not to disrupt your sleep, ever—OK, OK—they cannot promise this one. I promise not to give you puppy eyes every day and guilt you for that piece of food. I promise not to track my muddy paws all over the house. I promise not to shed fur all over the house. I promise not to give you heart palpitations when I run away.

I promise not to chew on furniture. I promise not to scratch the furniture, car, or boat. I promise not to do the Humpty dance with my neighborhood friends. This Tail A'la wishing promises list can go on forever, but you get the point.

SAMPLE WORKOUTS

A great example of a dog and owner workout is incorporating a daily morning routine focused on gratitude and mindfulness:

1. Begin with a brisk 5-minute walk to warm up, taking deep breaths and reflecting on what you're grateful for.

2. Inhale slowly and deeply through your nose, pause, and exhale through your mouth. Continue this breathing technique while walking for 15–30 minutes.
3. Conclude your workout with a 5-minute cooldown walk, wearing a smile on your face (smiling releases happy hormones).

If you have time, spend an additional 3–5 minutes in mindfulness by sitting quietly and petting your dog. Spending time in the fresh air will greatly benefit your health. This routine keeps you and your dog fit and strengthens the bond between the two of you through shared physical activity and thoughtful reflection.

Remember to bring water for both yourself and your dog, and monitor their energy levels to ensure a safe and enjoyable workout. Enjoy this routine, as it enhances your well-being and strengthens your connection with your furry friend.

EDUCATIONAL INSIGHTS

- Training Consistency: Encourage positive behavior and create a structured environment for your dog through consistent training.
- Socialization: Introduce your dog to different environments, people, and other animals to promote well-rounded social skills.
- Nutrition: Provide a balanced diet tailored to your dog's breed, age, and health requirements to ensure optimal health.
- Regular Checkups: Schedule periodic veterinary visits to monitor your dog's health and catch potential issues early.

- Mental Stimulation: Keep your dog engaged with puzzle toys, training exercises, and new experiences to stimulate their mind.

STORY

A win for the dog and boy. Imagine a young boy named Jonny who recently lost his father. Jonny felt lonely and withdrawn, struggling to find joy in his life. His mother adopted a dog named Pal, hoping it would help Jonny heal. From the moment Pal entered their home, he sensed Jonny's sorrow. Pal never left Jonny's side, offering comfort with gentle nudges and unwavering companionship. Gradually, Jonny began to smile again, finding solace in Pal's presence. The bond they formed became a source of emotional strength, demonstrating the profound impact a dog can have on healing and happiness.

RECOMMENDATIONS

- Discuss as a Family: Before adopting a dog, have a thorough discussion with your family about the responsibilities and commitments involved.
- Research Breeds: Consult various sources to find a breed that suits your family's lifestyle.
- Visit Shelters: Consider adopting dogs from shelters or rescue organizations to give them a second chance at a loving home.

- Prepare Your Home: Create a safe and welcoming environment for your new dog by providing essential supplies and a designated space.
- Schedule Training: Enroll in a training class to promote good behavior and strengthen your bond from the start.

SUMMARY

In summary, dog ownership brings great joy but comes with significant responsibilities. By committing to their care and understanding their needs, we cultivate a relationship filled with love, laughter, and mutual respect. As dog owners, we enrich our lives and provide our furry friends with the best possible care and companionship. As John Grogan, author of *Marley and Me*, once said, "A dog has no use for fancy cars, big homes, or designer clothes. A waterlogged stick will do just fine. A dog does not care if you are rich or poor, clever or dull, smart or dumb. Give him your heart, and he will give you his." This mutual commitment between the family and their dog will enhance everyone's lives.

CHAPTER 3

THE LITTER: THE JOURNEY OF RESPONSIBLE DOG OWNERSHIP

Taking a significant step into responsible and healthy dog ownership can present many challenges, especially with a puppy. This chapter focuses on being well-prepared for successful dog ownership. It will require patience—plenty of it—and the willingness to accept setbacks and failures. Training a dog, much like caring for a baby, takes time but can also be fun. Things may not go as planned, so stay positive, exercise self-control, forgive others, let go of the past, and keep moving forward. A well-thought-out plan that manages your expectations while incorporating injury prevention and cost-saving strategies will help you raise your puppy with love, appreciation, and patience.

HUMAN ELEMENT

According to the American Society for the Prevention of Cruelty to Animals (ASPCA), it is estimated that 78 million dogs are owned in the United States, representing 44 percent of all households. Sadly, 47 percent of those dogs are rehomed due to behavioral problems such as aggressive or problematic behavior. Additional reasons for dog surrender include housing restrictions or moving, financial strain from unexpected costs, and personal life changes. Given these statistics, it's crucial to consider all these factors seriously before embarking on the rollercoaster ride of dog ownership.

Mistakes and failures are common aspects of life as we face its challenges. It's important to acknowledge our shortcomings and view them as opportunities for growth. In the military, we learn that resilience can stem from failure, and success is not guaranteed. Annual training ensures that we adapt to changes and view stressful experiences as opportunities for learning. This helps us remain calm when chaos arises. Similarly, your response to your dog's mistakes will influence their learning and behavior. Patience and a cheerful outlook are key.

> It Happened to Me
>
> You ultimately get either a well-behaved dog, a slightly misbehaved one, or a crazy misfit hyena, depending on the level of involvement and time spent training and loving them. It's the age-old question of nature versus nurture. I think it's a combination of both—very diplomatic, I know.
>
> My parents, who are huge dog lovers, adopted an adorable pug puppy after their poodle passed away. There was only one concern: tons of shedding! My mom, a tidy person, was not used to this. After a few months, they had had enough of the hair all over the place, so they sought out another home for the sweet pug. The moral of the story is to make sure you complete all your homework before selecting your breed.

DOG CARE

Dogs reflect their owners' behaviors, a phenomenon explained by scientists through the concept of *mirror neurons*. These neurons, which are active in humans, are also believed to be found in dogs, allowing them to learn through observation.[4] Your dog will mirror this behavior if you remain calm and composed during stressful times. Additionally, dogs thrive on routines and consistent training. They are naturally optimistic, loving, and loyal, making them the perfect resilient companions to tackle life's challenges together.

When training your dog, expect setbacks, as they're part of the process. Just as a baby doesn't learn to walk overnight, your dog won't understand commands instantly. Growing, maturing, and training your dog requires significant dedication and effort. Be prepared for this and remember that your personal happiness and attitude will directly impact your dog's happiness and learning environment.

SAMPLE WORKOUTS

Canicross: A sport where a person and their dog run together, connected by an elastic leash

1. Warm-Up (10 minutes):
    - Take a light jog with your dog to get both of your hearts pumping.

---

[4] Fugazza, C., Andics, A., Magyari, L., Dror, S., Zempléni, A., and Miklósi, Á. "Rapid Learning of Object Names in Dogs." *Scientific Reports* 11, no. 1 (2021): 2222.

- Perform dynamic lunges to stretch and activate the larger muscles in your legs and back.

2. Main Workout (30 minutes):
    - Interval Running: Run for 2 minutes, then walk for 1 minute. Repeat 10 times.
    - Fetch Sprints: Throw a ball or flying disk and sprint with your dog to retrieve it.

3. Cooldown (10 minutes):
    - Walk slowly to gradually lower your heart rate.
    - Engage in gentle stretching exercises with your dog.

EDUCATIONAL INSIGHTS

- Patience is Key: Training takes time, and dogs learn best with consistent and patient guidance.
- Positive Reinforcement: Reward good behavior with treats, praise, and playtime.
- Routine is Essential: Dogs thrive on routine, so establish a consistent schedule for feeding, potty breaks, and exercise.
- Socialization: Introduce your dog to different environments, people, and other animals to help them become well-adjusted adult dogs.
- Health Checkups: Regular veterinary visits are crucial for monitoring your dog's health and identifying potential health problems early.
- Injury Prevention: Use proper equipment, avoid overexertion, and ensure safe play areas.

- Cost Savings: Invest in preventive care such as vaccinations and regular checkups to avoid costly emergencies later.

A NOTE ABOUT PERSEVERANCE FOR SUCCESS

Before we explore health and exercise, first and foremost, raise your white flag and surrender to past failures. Are you human? Yes, I hope so. Have you experienced failure at some point in your life? Yes, that's what being human is all about. Guess what? Your dogs may disappoint you too, but with time, training, and love, they can be well-behaved.

No matter the reason, it's all good. Ahh, doesn't it feel great to get that off your chest? All good. Forget past attempts or setbacks in improving your health—you're forgiven. It's human. Failures, when embraced, often lead to valuable lessons, knowledge, and new opportunities.

We all experience setbacks—it's a part of life. Don't be so hard on yourself. Not everything will go your way—get over it. No one is entitled to anything in life; you must work for and earn it. Success is never guaranteed—you need to work hard to earn respect. Stay true to your values, and good things and success will follow.

Failure is unavoidable and inevitable. Choose the growth mindset. The growth mindset enables individuals to continually improve and learn. This means having flexibility and creativity of thought, rather than being rigid and unimaginative. Like us, our dogs will often make mistakes, and we are responsible for guiding them. Be patient. Don't let them down. Those around you will observe your reactions after experiencing failure; manage it with grace. Take a deep breath—it's all good.

Our dogs will drive us insane at times, but we must remain calm. During stressful times, I encourage you to take 3-5 slow, deep breaths. This practice can help numerous physiological and neural systems in our body lower stress and cortisol levels, improve oxygen intake, increase focus and mindfulness, relax our bodies and muscles, and enhance our well-being and decision-making processes.

Another way our neural system interacts with our body and environment is through mirror neurons. Mirror neurons play a key role in how we learn behaviors and mannerisms through observation. They're especially active when we interact with our children, who closely watch, listen to, and imitate everything we do. It's no wonder that so many of you have a mini-me version of yourself—so darling! These are learned behaviors, and I bet our dogs are also watching, listening, and learning.

After each training event or mission, the military conducts an after-action review (AAR). Here's a brief description of the general process:

- Debrief: Analyze what occurred.
- Why did it occur?
- How can it be improved?
- Engage in an open discussion with your team or family.
- Create a summary or action plan to improve your next training or mission.

AFTER-ACTION REVIEW OF A PUPPY PEEING IN THE HOUSE:

Objective: Evaluate the incident where the puppy peed in the house to identify factors contributing to the behavior and apply strategies to prevent future occurrences.

Participants: Family members and anyone else who's caring for the puppy.

Discussion: Break down the incident into phases:

1. Before the incident: Discuss the circumstances that led to the accident. What signs did the puppy show to indicate it needed to go outside?
2. During the incident: Describe the actual moment the puppy peed indoors. What was happening at the time? Were there any distractions?
3. After the incident: Reflect on the actions taken immediately after the incident. How was the cleanup handled? What measures were implemented to prevent future incidents?

What went well:

- Recognizing that the puppy attempted to signal the need to go outside and noting what specific cues were observed
- Cleaning up the mess successfully.
- Acknowledging instances when the puppy successfully eliminated outside and identifying those cues.

Areas for improvement: Consider the factors that contributed to the incident, such as a lack of supervision or the failure to recognize and respond to the puppy's cues.

Review any recurring issues: Examine patterns that may indicate ongoing problems with the puppy regarding potty training.

Key lessons: Understand the puppy's body language and remain consistent and proactive in training to prevent accidents.

Action items: Create a clear and structured plan for your schedule, improve visuals focusing on the puppy, and enhance communication and responsibility among family members.

Documentation: Refer to the AAR as a reference to help the family train the puppy more effectively together.

This group participation enables your family to engage in a discovery session, express their opinions, identify and address any weaknesses or failures, and maintain what worked well. Sustain the good, discard the bad. Involve the entire family to ensure everyone has a voice. Freedom and collective bargaining are essential for organizing roles and responsibilities. Applying the AAR concept to the puppy peeing in the house allows you to systematically assess the incident, identify areas for improvement, and

> implement proactive measures to ensure successful potty training in the future.

STORY

Imagine you have just brought home a new puppy named Peach. She's adorable and full of energy and curiosity. On her first night, Peach had an accident in the living room. Instead of getting frustrated, you recall principles from this chapter. You calmly clean up the mess and take Peach outside, praising her when she does her business there. Over the next few weeks, you establish a consistent potty routine. While there are occasional accidents, you manage each with patience and persistence. Peach gradually learns, and your home becomes a happier place for both of you.

Your happiness will have a direct correlation to the joy shared with your dog. Learn from your failures, embrace them, and learn valuable lessons from them; it will happen. A cheerful outlook can create a more positive learning environment for your dog. Dogs genuinely care about our happiness and strive to make us happy. If you keep a positive mindset, who knows? You may be as resilient as your dog.

Our dogs are optimistic, loving, and loyal, making them resilient companions for tackling life's challenges together. Our dogs don't judge us and will love you for who you are, regardless of the time you can spend with them. Everyone occasionally falls off the horse, but it's our dedication to get back on that matters.

Exercise is not just about physical fitness; it's a key to a cheerful outlook and overall well-being for humans and dogs. We all have our reasons for not exercising, but it's time to own them and learn from them. Let's not forget our furry friends who can also benefit from our active lifestyle.

As a physical therapist (PT), I have heard every excuse in the book for avoiding exercise—trust me. Here are some common excuses people have given me, including what your dog might think:

Common Human Excuses:	Your Dog is Thinking:
"I didn't exercise because _____ (insert excuse)" It's a small setback. Take ownership of your decisions.	What about me? Is it time to have fun yet?
I'm too busy and don't have time.	Get off your bum. I saw you hit the snooze button twice this morning!
I'm just too tired and don't have the energy.	(Drooling) I see you eating that filet mignon, and I want some!
I don't have any motivation.	Get off your caboose—choo choo! Canicross, buddy—I will lead you!
I get bored easily.	Dog'ercise with me, mi amigo!
I really don't feel like sweating, taking another shower, and getting ready again.	You're beautiful, inside and out. Now get your sweat and sexy on!

I struggle with low self-esteem. I don't want to be embarrassed and judged by others.	From what I can see, you look dog darn good in the bathroom (see above). Everyone will be looking at me anyway—let's be real! *Woof!*
Exercise is not fun.	You're doing the wrong exercise plan. Let's 'Dog'ercise with the tips and ideas in this book, and it'll be tail-wagging fun—just wait and see!
Insert any other excuse	I just want to play and have fun!

TIP #2
NEVER MAKE EXCUSES.
EMBRACE FAILURES.

RECOMMENDATIONS

- Research: Understand the specific needs of your dog's breed.
- Plan: Create a training schedule and commit to following it consistently.
- Patience: Embrace a cheerful outlook and practice patience.
- Exercise: Make sure to include daily exercise routines for you and your dog.
- Routine: Create regular routines for feeding, potty breaks, and training.

- Prevent Injuries: Use appropriate equipment and ensure play areas are safe.
- Save Money: Invest in preventive care, such as vaccinations and regular checkups, to avoid costly emergencies.

SUMMARY

Becoming a responsible dog owner is a journey filled with challenges and rewards. Your most valuable tools are patience, consistency, and a positive, cheerful outlook. Embrace the process, learn from setbacks, and cherish your dog's unconditional love and companionship. You can ensure a healthier and more affordable experience by integrating injury prevention and cost-saving measures. As Lao Tzu said, "The journey of a thousand miles begins with a single step." Take that step with confidence and a wagging tail. Enjoy with happiness.

CHAPTER 4

HONESTY AND OPPORTUNITY: THE PATH TO HEALTH AND BONDING

Injury prevention is crucial for maintaining a healthy and active lifestyle for humans and dogs. Incorporating effective exercise routines with your dog can help reduce medical and veterinary expenses. Embracing honesty about your physical activity and health habits will ensure that both you and your dog receive the best possible care. This proactive approach can help you avoid injuries, enhance overall well-being, and deepen the bond with your furry friend.

Gather the necessary ingredients to support your growth. As we know, water is just one of the essential ingredients needed for a seed to grow. For puppies and babies, that crucial ingredient is milk. The nutrients in the milk are essential for our growth and development. To thrive, you need to *get the milk*. If you're missing ingredients, it'll be difficult to grow. Be upfront about which ingredients you're missing. Once you realize this, look for opportunities to plant and grow. It begins with you and your dog, who's looking up to you. Remember Tip #2: Make no excuses and embrace failures. You're now learning the key elements and how these tips will provide you with the mindset and framework. You need to provide these essential factors to your physical therapist (PT) so that we can help you.

HUMAN ELEMENT

Honesty is paramount in physical therapy. Being truthful with your PT about your activities and any challenges allows for a more personalized and effective treatment plan. Your PT helps you stay active, pain-free, and maintain strong muscles and bones.

Ideally, you'll respond truthfully about your progress, allowing your PT to determine your best course of action. If the patient comes in and says, "I haven't had time to do the exercises because of XYZ," or, "This movement is painful, so I've avoided all the exercises." A good PT will appreciate your honesty and adjust your plan accordingly. Don't admit to doing exercises when you haven't. If you do this, your PT will be unable to adjust your care plan in a way that will make a more meaningful and quicker impact on your goals. It's always better to tell the truth.

The PT can help develop additional strategies for your home program. We don't judge; we want to help you. When your PT asks for information, this is your chance to share details that can support your progress, ideally leading to less pain and faster recovery. A lack of essential elements, such as valuable information, will hinder your recovery.

DOG CARE

Dogs also thrive on honesty and consistent care. Just as you need proper nutrition and activities to grow and stay healthy, your dog does too. Being honest about your dog's health and exercise routine helps you create a better plan to keep them fit and happy. Exercising with your dog improves their physical health but also deepens your bond. Exercise with your dog not only benefits their physical health but also strengthens the bond between you. Dogs that exercise with their owners are often happier and healthier, creating a win-win situation for both of you.

Just as we do in the military, set a *checkpoint* for yourself to serve as your barometer. It's a momentary snapshot that may vary throughout the day: Are you happy or sad? How is your energy level? How well are you sleeping? How are your nutrition and overall health? You get the idea. Your *baseline* can be measured subjectively in your mood, stress levels, energy levels, or objectively in your resting heart rate, blood pressure, body weight, or measures of motion and strength.

Many smartwatches can provide a wealth of health information to track over time. I highly recommend you track what makes sense to you. Know your body's baseline and be mindful of your dog's as well. Their wagging tail easily measures your dog's happiness. Being aware of both yourself and your dog can help you recognize when you need an extra push, a hug, better sleep, or a healthier diet. When all systems function in harmony, we call this *optimization*.

To accomplish this, take a moment to slow down and identify the unwanted noise you want to block out—be honest. You must be truthful with yourself and don't hesitate to seek guidance when needed—there's no problem with that. We refer to this as being mission-ready, actively seeking advice, and exploring new opportunities. Many people feel they lack time to exercise, but is the real issue that we don't use our time effectively, which many of us fall victim to? Guess what? Your expiration term of service is a military term used to denote the completion of a contract. Think of your old contract as expired; you're starting fresh with a new one. *Ruff!* Let's find more ways to be efficient while including our dogs. WILCO (will comply) *Ruff! Ruff!*

SAMPLE WORKOUTS

Dog'ercise is a fun and effective way to incorporate regular physical activity into your routine with your dog. This routine helps both of you stay fit while also offering quality bonding time.

1. Warm-Up: Get on the floor to play with or pet your dog.
2. Strength Training: Incorporate bodyweight exercises like squats, lunges, and push-ups while using your dog's favorite toy to keep them engaged.
3. Cardiovascular training: Run up and down the stairs repeatedly or jog with your dog for 10–15 minutes.
4. Cooldown: Take a slow walk and gently stretch to help you and your dog recover.

Upon closer examination, it became clear to experts that dog responsibilities are a common and significant barrier preventing people from exercising. Dog lovers—light bulb moment! I'll admit, I didn't understand it at first because I use my time with my dogs to help me stay active. I also know I'm not normal—I can't sit still, and it feels weird. I wondered why other people weren't active with their dogs. Is it due to a lack of time or a lack of understanding about the importance of movement? Or, even worse, could walking the dog lead to injuries that prevent people from being active? Let's use our dog responsibilities to teach others how to move safely. It's a responsible use of one's time and a win-win. There's so much bonding; those who work out together stick together.

EDUCATIONAL INSIGHTS

- Be truthful with your medical provider about your health and activity levels.
- Make sure your dog exercises regularly to help prevent health issues.
- Exercising with your dog strengthens your bond and improves both your well-being.
- Incorporate physical activity into your daily routine to support a healthier lifestyle.

STORY

Maria, a patient, struggled to fit exercise into her busy schedule while managing her responsibilities as a dog owner. She was upfront with her PT, who recommended combining her dog's exercise routine with her own and reading *Healthy Living with Your Dog: 21 Tips for a Healthy, Injury-Free Life*. Maria started Dog'ercising and saw significant improvements in both her health and her dog's happiness. They became a fitter, closer duo, and Maria discovered how honesty and creativity could help overcome obstacles.

Now imagine Sarah, a busy professional who loves her dog, Max. She often skips her exercise routine, claiming she doesn't have time. Her PT suggested combining her workouts with Max's walks to make the most of her time. Sarah starts jogging with Max and practicing strength exercises in the park. This new routine helped Sarah recover more quickly and established healthy baselines and checkpoints for both of them. Sarah feels happier, healthier, and more connected to her beloved dog, showing how honesty and innovation can transform lives.

Pearls of Wisdom: If you're not satisfied with your PT, don't hesitate to ask for someone who may be a better fit for you; there's nothing wrong with that. Many of us are too polite to speak up because we do not want to hurt anyone's feelings. I'm here to say that it happens more often than you think—if a patient is unhappy with their progress, doesn't share the same sense of humor, or, in the worst case, feels the care is poor and doesn't see any value in the visit. You should be able to enjoy physical therapy if that's your style, and you should feel comfortable having honest conversations built on trust with your healthcare providers.

HOW TO ASK FOR A CHANGE OF PROVIDER

HERE ARE A FEW EXAMPLES:

- "I love what we've done together so far, but I feel that working with another PT would be the best way to reach my goals. Who would you recommend helping me back on the pickleball court?"
- "I haven't seen as much progress as I had hoped for this in this timeline. Would you recommend a colleague with more experience in treating this diagnosis for a second opinion?

- Or, often simply asking, "Let's bring in another provider to collaborate—who would you recommend?" can be helpful.

There is no one-size-fits-all approach. As I tell my patients, we're all wired and built differently. As a healthcare consumer, you have a right to find the best provider who best suits your needs. As healthcare providers, we are responsible for acting in our best interests using research, experience, and specific needs to guide our decisions. Sometimes, things just don't click, and that's OK. Do not let this discourage you—be your own health advocate. The same is true when choosing that perfect breed for your family pet or finding the right veterinarian to keep your dog healthy. Sometimes, choosing a puppy from a litter is love at first sight. Sometimes, your gut—or spouse—tells you to keep looking. You never know where you'll find that perfect companion—it may be at the local shelter, a rescue organization, or a breeder of your choice. If you follow the dog's family oath, there'll be unlimited doggy licks and kisses.

RECOMMENDATIONS

- Be honest with your physical therapist about your activity levels and challenges you're facing.
- Incorporate your dog's exercise needs into your own fitness routine.
- Track your progress and adjust your plan when necessary.
- Look for opportunities to stay active and healthy with your dog.
- Don't hesitate to switch healthcare providers if you feel it's not a good fit.

SUMMARY

Always keep your eyes open. Your dog's eyes are always on, waiting for a chance to spend time together. They crave the opportunity and time with you. Embracing transparency and creativity in your fitness routines with your dog can lead to improved health, a deeper bond, and a more fulfilling life. Remember, every decision you make is a step toward a healthier, happier journey for both you and your dog. The more honest you are with yourself, the more you will experience life's riches. Opportunities will come your way, and when they do, keep those floodgates open and let them flow. Opportunity is all around us. Every decision you make is a drop of water guiding you along your journey. Grab your surfboard or bring your dog on a raft and ride that wild river together. I promise you, it'll be a fun and exciting ride!

TIP #3
BE HONEST. SEEK OPPORTUNITIES.

CHAPTER 5

PAWS AND FEET: MOVING TOWARD BETTER HEALTH TOGETHER

Exercise is essential for a healthy life, offering benefits that go far beyond physical fitness. Various levels of exercise intensity result in different levels of perspiration (a.k.a. sweating) as your body attempts to cool itself down due to increased physical activity. This is known as thermoregulation—a fancy word for maintaining body temperature—essentially your body's thermostat. That's why you'll see numerous reminders about the importance of proper hydration as activity levels increase.

Regular physical activity can help prevent injuries, elevate mood, enhance cognitive function, reduce stress, strengthen muscles, and help combat memory loss. The best part is that you don't need a gym membership or to break a sweat to enjoy these benefits. Just like dogs naturally do, incorporating exercise into your daily routine can help prevent injuries, maintain overall well-being, and reduce healthcare costs. Plus, exercise is great for you—it's the cherry on top! As physical therapists, we use it to combat any pain or discomfort you may experience.

Sweating is great, and I encourage it once you build up to a solid workout. However, you don't need to sweat to call it exercise. Truth. Our dogs don't sweat—you'll learn more about this later.

HUMAN ELEMENT

Being honest about what prevents you from staying active is crucial to living a healthier life. Our dogs show honesty in their behavior every day. By reflecting on your habits, behaviors, and distractions, and observing your dog's mannerisms, you can increase your awareness and make better choices for a more active lifestyle.

Finding the energy for exercise can be challenging, but using your time more efficiently can help you build a routine that works for you. Prioritize activities that bring you happiness and health. As we age, it's important to maintain a healthy body and mind to fully enjoy life. We all have areas where we could be more efficient; acknowledging this can help us make the most of our time. Consider tracking your activities for a week. Take note of how much time you spend on each activity. If you notice wasted time, how can you better allocate it?

Life can be chaotic, but focusing on simple and necessary actions can make it easier to navigate. Just like dogs, who find joy in simple things, we can benefit from focusing on what truly matters. Everyone is an athlete because even the smallest movements require some athleticism.

To live a healthier life, be honest with yourself about what limitations affect your activity level. At times, finding the motivation to exercise can be truly difficult. Managing your time efficiently will help you build a routine that works for you, while using it effectively will provide you with the flexibility and freedom to decide how to spend your free time. Life happens, and things come up like they always do. Prioritize what brings happiness and well-being. Maintaining a healthy body and mind is crucial for reaping the benefits of your hard work as you age.

I often overthink tasks that could be completed quickly, like writing an email. However, when I need to purchase plane tickets for an upcoming trip, I book them promptly to get them out of my mind. Some of you may do the opposite. The point is, we all have time in our lives when we could be more efficient. Hopefully, it's clear by now that life will always have its crazy moments due to society's demands.

DOG CARE

Dogs don't sweat. Panting is the primary method for maintaining body temperature, which increases the risk of heat-related injuries during heightened activity. Providing a constant source of water will keep them active and happy, no matter the level of activity. This reminds us that exercise doesn't have to be intense to be beneficial. They find joy in movement and simplicity—and we can too. Including our dogs in our exercise routines helps us build a consistent and enjoyable path to better health.

Dogs hold us accountable and inspire us to stay active. Their enthusiasm is contagious, making exercise both enjoyable and rewarding. Moving together, you and your dog can improve your health and fitness. Why is that? Just look at our furry friends—most are living carefree, joyful lives, simply happy every day, especially when they see you coming through that door. The joy and excitement of walking into the house never gets old for them, whether you've been gone for 15 minutes or 8 hours. It never gets old, does it? When we're provided with the essentials of life, such as water, food, and shelter, there's nothing to worry about. The world may be complex, but at our core, we're no different from our dogs. We need the basics, not the complicated; simplicity works if you let it.

> KISS PRINCIPLE: Keep it simple, silly!

So how do we keep it simple? The answer is so easy, it'll blow your mind. If you're reading this, you're an athlete—yes, everyone! While we all have a competitive spirit in some way, some of us are more athletic than others. If you look up the word "athlete," you'll find it defined as someone involved in sports or demonstrating exceptional physical ability. Did you get out of your bed to stand up today? Walk to get the mail? Take the stairs today or squat to pick something up? My friends, if you've done even one of these, you are an athlete. Why? Because movement itself requires athleticism, and some activities simply demand more than others. It's true. Our daily activities rely on our muscles working together efficiently, whether it is catching a ball or brushing our teeth. This coordination helps us achieve multiple daily goals.

SAMPLE WORKOUTS

Here are twenty everyday activities that require athleticism and can be done with your dog—no gym membership is required:
- Squats: Sit down and stand up from a chair (try without using armrests)
- Lunges while walking down the hallway
- Hip hinge to pick something up (similar to a Romanian deadlift)

- Improve balance by folding laundry while standing on one leg
- Plank variations during commercial breaks or while playing with your dog
- Repeatedly walking or running up and down stairs
- Hold a static squat or lunge while brushing teeth
- Stand on your toes while washing the dishes
- Throw a ball and squat to greet your dog between each toss
- Park farther away to add more steps to your day
- Stay active by mopping, sweeping, and dusting
- Walk your shopping cart back to the return area
- Do push-ups against a wall or on the floor
- Work in your garden or water your plants
- Cook meals while dancing to your favorite tune
- Take the stairs instead of the elevator
- Do yard work, such as shoveling or raking leaves
- Do jumping jacks intermittently throughout the day
- Hold static lunges or squats for a set amount of time
- Engage in various activities with your dog

I know—I just keep blowing your mind and unlocking all that hidden potential! Opening your eyes to the many athletic movements you incorporate into your daily life feels great. Potential (stored) energy transforms into kinetic (moving) energy, powering movement for both us and our dogs. Do you remember watching that puppy grow from one year old to two years old? As our dogs explore the outdoors or learn to jump onto the couch or bed, they need both power and coordination. Each increasingly challenging task requires greater athleticism, control, and balance.

From infancy to where you are today, you've become a resilient athlete—some of us with more scars than others. We have each challenged our bodies in different ways and shaped ourselves into various types of athletes. I remind my seasoned and older athletes that the activities they've put their bodies through over the years naturally lead to scars and wear and tear. Nothing is wrong with that—it's a sign of life well-lived, complete with battle wounds. Pursuing dreams and enjoyment—we all have potential and are all athletes. Enough said, my mover and shaker.

When we embrace the idea of movement and athleticism, what do our daily activities become? If you're following along, you're right—exercise. Every movement you make throughout the day is exercise, just like your dog. Now, if you incorporate a *consistent* daily or weekly exercise routine with your furry companion, you'll be on your way to better health and fitness in no time, one paw and step at a time.

See the connection? Your dog's companionship will hold both of you accountable to each other. The movement in your daily activities, along with your dog's, helps you stay active throughout the day. Recognizing and embracing this fact will help you stay committed more often. As a responsible dog owner—and I know you are—this is the one task I ask of you. You can answer the questions below as you go through the book or wait until you've finished reading it. You're in charge!

EDUCATIONAL INSIGHTS

Dogs naturally incorporate exercise into their daily lives, showing us that movement is both essential and enjoyable. By following their examples, we can incorporate more movement into our routines, improving both our health and our dogs' well-being.

In the military, choices are not always optional. We learn about courses of action (COAs) to guide decision-making. As the commander of this book, your assigned COA is to complete these questions. That's an order. Grab your mighty ink sword. Set realistic goals that you can commit to. Use the 21 Tips to uncover guiding principles that will keep you moving forward with your dog:

- Opportunities for Improvement (Tip #2: Embrace and Learn): What exercise habits did you previously try with your dog that didn't work? What do you think were the reasons for their failures?
- Current Barriers (Tip #3: Be Honest): What prevents you from being active with your dog?
- Goals (Tip #3: Seek Opportunities): What fitness goals do you want to achieve with your dog?

    - Daily goals:
    - Weekly goals:
    - Monthly goals:

- Action Plan (Tip #4: Execute an Action Plan): Write down your plan to get active.
- Pack Involvement (Tip #5: Support Your Pack): Who could help unite the pack and enjoy being a part of it? Invite them in!
- Visualization (Tip #4: Visualize Success): Write down a few strategies you'll commit to in order to keep your action plan on track and accomplish your mission, such as, "I will create a daily mantra to repeat to myself," "I will write in

a journal daily," "I will place a sticky note reminder on my bathroom mirror," or "I will set a daily reminder on my phone." Check out www.movebettertogether.com for a companion worksheet that will help you.

Mantra to maintain momentum when you're in motion:

_____

Mantra for when you're exhausted and unmotivated (push through):

_____

A fun daily mantra to remind you of your commitment to your friend (insert your dog's name):

_____

Use the tactics that work for you and discard the rest—you're the captain.

As Tony Robbins once said, "If you envision your goals, write them out to bring them to life." It is the visualization process that many successful people live by." Now close your eyes (seriously) and imagine a specific scene or picture that reflects your self-worth and where you would like to be. Have your dog sit with you and do it together—it'll be fun!

The law of attraction states that your thoughts and beliefs shape your reality. There is some scientific evidence that the neurons in your brain and body influence decision-making and draw you toward what attracts you. Try this technique at bedtime to reinforce those neurons and help them become embedded in your memory. Use this to your advantage, letting your visualization guide the way like a torch lighting your path. It will also keep you more connected to the outcome and engaged during the process.

Writing down how often you want to be reminded of your action plan can help you establish a routine that reinforces your vision. My studies in neurology during graduate school may have instilled this skill and inspired me to further pursue it. It's the study of your nerves, your brain, and how they work together to communicate inside your body. I guess they "neuromuscled" me—*da-dum—crash*! Who knows? For example, I write reminders on sticky notes and place them where I will see them daily, such as the bathroom mirror, my calendar, my laptop, or even the pop-up notes section on my screen. Feel my energy?

STORY

One day, Jane realized her sedentary lifestyle was impacting her health. Inspired by her energetic dog, Will, she decided to make a change. She and Will began each day with a walk around the block, gradually increasing their distance. They played fetch, practiced agility, and even danced together in the living room. Jane not only lost weight and became healthier, but she also strengthened her bond with Will. They became a team, encouraging each other to stay active and happy.

Imagine coming home exhausted after a long day at work, with no energy left for exercise—until your dog, full of enthusiasm, brings you the leash. Their excitement inspires you to find the energy for a short walk. That walk turns into a jog, leaving you both feeling invigorated. This simple act of moving together lifts your mood and deepens your bond with your dog. It's a reminder that even on the toughest days, our dogs inspire us to keep moving.

Our dogs are the best listeners you could ask for. Give it a try—you'll see. I promise.

RECOMMENDATIONS

- Reflect on past exercise routines with your dog and identify why they didn't work.
- List current obstacles preventing you from being active with your dog.
- Set daily, weekly, and monthly fitness goals for you and your dog.
- Develop a clear action plan to achieve these goals.
- Involve family, friends, and neighbors in your fitness journey.
- Use visualization techniques to stay motivated and committed to your action plan.
- Create daily mantras or affirmations to keep yourself inspired.
- Place reminders in visible places to stay on track with your goals.

SUMMARY

Exercise is essential for both humans and dogs. By incorporating simple movements into your daily routine and engaging with your dog, you can improve your health and strengthen your bond. Remember, as another saying goes, "Every great and wonderful journey begins with the first small move forward." With your dog by your side, each step becomes more enjoyable.

TIP #4
EXECUTE AN ACTION PLAN.
VISUALIZE SUCCESS.

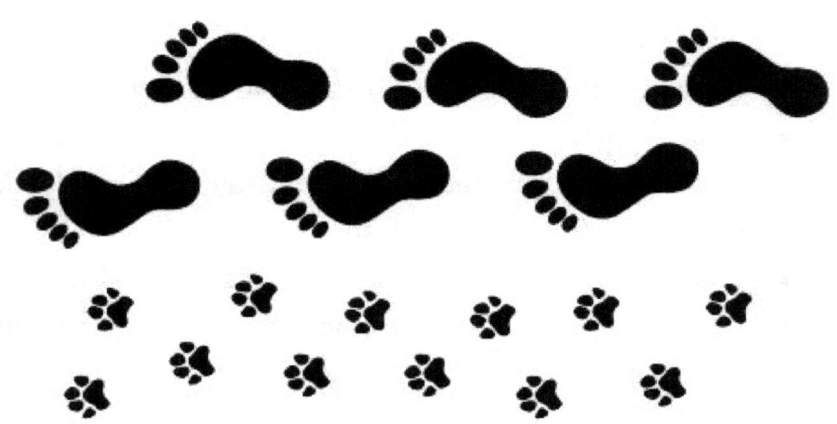

CHAPTER 6

RUFF AND READY: EXERCISING WITH YOUR PACK FOR A HEALTHIER LIFE

Injury prevention isn't just about avoiding physical harm; it's about protecting your well-being, reducing healthcare costs, and preserving long-term quality of life. Regular exercise with your dog helps you achieve these goals while deepening the bond with your furry companion.

HUMAN ELEMENT

Regular exercise offers numerous benefits for humans. Physically active individuals typically live an average of seven years longer than those who are inactive. Exercise is a crucial tool for mental health, reducing the risk of depression by 20–30 percent—even just ten minutes of physical activity can lift your mood. It also significantly reduces the risk of falls in older adults by 30 percent by improving balance and strengthening bone density. For children, physical activity is linked to improved academic performance.[5] Incorporating regular exercise into

---

[5] Lee, I. M., and Shiroma, E. J. "Physical Activity and Life Expectancy." *Journal of the American Medical Association* 312, no. 3 (2014): 206-208.

your daily routine is a proactive way to tackle challenges and enhance your overall well-being. This book provides a comprehensive overview of the benefits of exercising with dogs, enabling humans to exercise together, improve their family's quality of life, have fun, and stay active as a unit. I call this wrestling with the pack.

You and your companion are the pack. If your family is larger, then you have a larger pack. If your pack is against you, it will be hard to navigate the world—uff-da (that's Scandinavian for "Oh no!")! When your pack is united, the world is yours to explore. You should always work to get the pack together and make a pack—pun intended. *Ruff!* Let's not treat this like a typical New Year's resolution where you vow to get in shape, lose weight, or adopt a healthier habit, only to lose your momentum. That can feel overwhelming—like a bowl of hotdish spilling over the edges. A Midwest thing—you betcha! It isn't meant to be, but it's the doggy truth. Most of us know what we should be doing to live and eat healthy, right?

It involves eating nutritious foods in the right portions, incorporating a variety of colorful foods, getting enough sleep, and staying active. It's the light switch that can be difficult to turn on and make a lifestyle choice when it's easy to hit the fast food chains or rest after a long day of work. No matter what your sport, activity, or life choices are, without improving and maintaining our health, we will inevitably hit a pothole—if we're lucky—versus a roadblock, or worse, a grave site. Everyone needs to prepare for battle. Every. Single. Day.
Repeat this mantra:

Nourish my body,
move my soul;
in balance with daily battles,
I find my whole.

Despite our vulnerabilities, there is no magic dog bone or miracle pill for our health—no matter what you want to believe, what the latest gimmicks suggest, or what you may have heard. It's all about the movement.

To summarize, consider these eye-opening statistics that'll motivate you:

- Physically active people live an average of seven years longer than those who are inactive.[6]
- Adults who engage in regular exercise have a 20–30 percent lower risk of developing depression.[7]
- Regular physical activity can reduce the risk of falls in older adults by 30 percent[8] and can lower the risk of osteoporosis later in life by enhancing bone mass, especially when engaged in physical activity during childhood.[9]
- Just 10 minutes of exercise can improve your mood.[10]
- Children who engage in regular physical activity show improved cognitive function and better academic performance.[11]

---

[6] Lee and Shiroma, "Physical Activity," 206-208.

[7] Craft, L. L., and Perna, F. M. "The Benefits of Exercise for the Clinically Depressed." *The Primary Care Companion to The Journal of Clinical Psychiatry* 6, no. 3 (2004): 104-111.

[8] World Health Organization.

[9] Sherrington, C., Tiedemann, A., Fairhall, N. J., et al. "Exercise to Prevent Falls in Older Adults: An Updated Systematic Review and Meta-Analysis." *British Journal of Sports Medicine* 45, no. 6 (2011): 344-352.

[10] Damrongthai, C., et al. "Acute Effects of 10-Minute Running on Mood and Cognitive Function." *Scientific Reports* 11, no. 1 (2021): 12096; Basso, J. C., and Suzuki, W. A. "The Effects of Acute Exercise on Mood, Cognition, Neurophysiology, and Neurochemical Pathways: A Review." *Brain Plasticity* 4, no. 1 (2018): 23-38.

[11] Donnelly, J. E., and Lambourne, K. "Classroom Physical Activity Breaks and Academic Performance." *Preventive Medicine* 52, suppl. 1 (2011): S36-S42.

With that in mind, it's about intentionally taking action and striving to be the best version of yourself. Every choice you make shapes your path—remember the law of attraction. By making positive choices for yourself, your dog, and your pack, the clearest path will unfold before you. That's the lifestyle. One person can create a ripple that grows into a tidal wave of change. That's right—it only takes one brave leader to inspire and guide the pack.

There's no secret sauce, as they say. This is not David versus Goliath or an intense showdown like Big Red versus Old Yeller. It's about making small, consistent choices that lead to a stronger, more unified pack. Everyone wins when the whole pack is involved—even if it's just you and your dog. Like anything in life, with practice, effort, and challenge, adaptation happens over time; consistency is key. Just like training a top athlete or a champion show dog, change takes time. Get the pack involved, stay active together, and make this world a better place. So, wrestle with the pack, lead the pack, and grow the pack! That's a big 10–4, meaning yes, OK, understood, affirmative, or you betcha! Lima Charlie (loud and clear)!

DOG CARE

Like humans, dogs greatly benefit from regular exercise. It helps maintain a healthy weight, reduces the risk of chronic diseases, and enhances mental well-being. Regular physical activity keeps your dog healthy, happier, and less prone to behavioral issues. Exercising together deepens the bond between you and your dog, fostering a strong and harmonious pack.

SAMPLE WORKOUTS

Remember, Dog'ercise is any fun and interactive workout you can enjoy with your dog.

1. Start with a 10-minute warm-up of brisk walking or jogging. Notice a theme? Repetition is key.
2. Next, incorporate exercises like walking on various terrains to strengthen your balance muscles. Try grass, hills, gravel roads, or hiking trails.
3. Engage in activities like throwing a ball and sprinting or walking to retrieve it. Try an obstacle course with hurdles and cones.
4. Finish with a cooldown of gentle walking and stretching. This routine gives you a full-body workout while keeping your dog engaged and active.

EDUCATIONAL INSIGHTS

- Consistency is Key: Regular exercise is more effective than occasional intense workouts.
- Hydration: Make sure your dog always has fresh water before, during, and after exercise.
- Breed Considerations: Every breed has unique exercise needs, so customize your routine to match your dog's breed and energy level.
- Watch for Signs: Observe your dog's cues—if they seem tired or distressed, it's time to take a break.

- Vet Visits: Routine veterinary checkups help ensure your dog is healthy and ready for exercise.

STORY

Imagine a family rescuing a dog named Duke. Initially shy and fearful, Duke gained confidence and energy through regular Dog'ercise sessions. The family also experienced improvements in their physical fitness and overall mood. Their daily exercise routine became a cherished family tradition, highlighting the transformative power of shared movement.

Picture this: Katie, a busy professional, feels disconnected from her family and her energetic dog, Rocket. She begins a daily Dog'ercise routine and soon notices stronger family connections, a happier Rocket, and significantly decreased stress levels. This newfound harmony highlights the importance of exercising together, promoting both emotional and physical well-being.

RECOMMENDATIONS

- Schedule Daily Exercise: Establish a daily routine that includes at least 30 minutes of physical activity for both you and your dog.
- Mix Activities: Vary your exercises to keep them exciting and engaging for both you and your dog.
- Track Progress: Keep a journal to monitor your and your dog's progress, noting improvements in both your fitness and your dog's mood.

- Engage with the Community: Join local dog-walking groups or fitness classes to stay motivated and connect with like-minded individuals.
- Educate Yourself: Continuously learn best practices for exercising with your dog and stay informed about new activities and tips.

SUMMARY

Nourish my body, move my soul; in balance with daily battles, I find my whole.

Prioritizing exercise for both you and your dog leads to a healthier, happier, and more connected life. Embrace the journey, support your pack, and lead with consistency and compassion.

TIP #5
SUPPORT YOUR PACK.
INCREASE GOODNESS.

CHAPTER 7

HEALTHY HABITS FOR YOU AND YOUR DOG

Maintaining a healthy lifestyle with proper nutrition, regular exercise, and adequate sleep can help prevent health issues and lower medical costs. Experts agree that adopting a healthy lifestyle could significantly reduce the need for many healthcare services. In fact, many healthcare professionals acknowledge that if everyone ate nutritious foods, got enough sleep, exercised regularly, and stayed hydrated, their jobs might become obsolete. Through my many conversations with physicians and other medical providers over the years, a clear consensus has emerged. In summary, taking care of your body's basic needs helps mitigate your risk of injury. It is really no mystery to solve, and as Scooby-Doo might say, "Ruh–roh!"

HUMAN ELEMENT

A healthy gut microbiome—a term referring to the beneficial bacteria in our digestive system—is essential for overall well-being. While processed foods can disrupt its delicate balance, nutritious foods can help support and strengthen it. To maintain this balance, incorporate routine resets, such as adjusting your diet. Reset means recalibrating yourself—pausing, reflecting, and returning to your desired self. Just like rebooting a computer can resolve issues, a nutritional reset can optimize your body's performance. When your computer freezes, a hard restart is often the only solution—think of this as a reset. The computer shuts down, reboots (hopefully), and functions as it should. Just like prayer and meditation help people reset, taking a hard pause allows you to restart and move forward with clarity.

What does that mean? Think of it as resetting your nutritional intake. You eliminate unhealthy stuff (i.e., sugar, excess carbs, alcohol, and desserts) and put well-balanced and colorful foods into your body. Be sure to consult a healthcare professional or registered dietitian before making significant changes to your diet. They should be able to provide personalized advice based on your specific health needs and goals. Make sure to read well-regarded books on healthy nutrition, backed by evidence, to help guide your decisions.

In life, there is a healthy balance of nutritious foods (such as colorful vegetables and fruit) versus indulgences (desserts, sugary drinks, etc.) for our body. The greater sum should be in favor of good, healthy days. I'm not a nutritional expert, nor claim to be, but it's okay to stray from time to time and savor the wonders of the world. That's called fun—just ask your belly and taste buds. You just need that balance. I love desserts and sweets, especially chocolate. It's my weakness, for sure. I know this, so I ensure I make sure to bank my good days and reward myself with chocolate from time to time. Not every day. The same applies to your dog. You don't give your dog daily frosty treats because they're unhealthy (and expensive!). We know all this.

DOG CARE

Like humans, dogs thrive with a healthy microbiome. Proper nutrition fuels their bodies, helping them to perform their best. Creating an appropriate exercise regimen for your dog requires considering their breed, age, health, size, and energy level. Customizing activities ensures they stay healthy and happy. Consulting a veterinarian can help you create a suitable exercise plan.

You may wonder why there aren't specific activity guidelines for aerobic and strength training for dogs. That is because, depending on the governing body consulted, there are between 195 and over 300 breeds of dogs, each varying in size and shape. Environmental factors must be considered, whether you live in a cold or hot climate. And here you thought that there were only 101 Dalmatians—wrong! That's a lot of breeds, eh? It's enough to make Lassie turn her head and never come home. Let's get a *woof! woof!* from the big dogs or a *yip! yip!* from my smaller fellas.

Customizing your dog's exercise routine to tailor it to their specific needs and requirements is crucial. Here are some general guidelines to help you determine the right amount of exercise for your dog:

- Consider Breed Characteristics: Different breeds have unique energy levels and exercise needs. Research your dog's breed to understand their natural tendencies. For example, high-energy breeds like vizslas may require more mental and physical stimulation than lower-energy breeds, such as basset hounds.
- Age Matters: Puppies experience bursts of energy but also need plenty of rest for healthy growth and development.

As dogs age, their activity levels tend to decline, so it's essential to adjust the intensity and duration of exercise accordingly. Senior dogs often benefit from gentler activities.

- Health Check: Consult your veterinarian before starting or changing your dog's exercise routine. Health conditions like arthritis or heart issues can affect the type and amount of exercise they can handle. A vet's guidance is crucial for creating a safe and suitable plan.
- Size and Weight: Larger dogs often require more exercise to burn energy and maintain a healthy weight. Smaller breeds may require less intense activity but still benefit from mental stimulation. Overweight dogs might need a gradual increase in activity as they build strength and improve fitness.
- Individual Variability: Dogs have unique energy levels and preferences like humans. Observe your dog's cues and adjust their exercise routine accordingly. Some may thrive on high-energy activities, while others prefer gentle walks or playtime.
- Mix It Up: Keep your dog engaged and prevent boredom by incorporating a variety of activities, such as walks, runs, interactive play, and mentally stimulating games. These are just as important as physical exercise for their overall well-being.
- Duration and Frequency: Introduce exercise gradually and increase intensity over time. Focus on regular, consistent activity rather than occasional intense sessions. The ideal duration and frequency depend on your dog's needs, but a good starting point is often 30 minutes to 2 hours a day, spread across various activities.

- Watch for Signs of Fatigue or Discomfort: Monitor your dog's behavior during and after exercise. If they show signs of fatigue, limping, or discomfort, adjust the routine accordingly and consult your vet if necessary.

SAMPLE WORKOUTS

Include both aerobic and strength-building exercises in your routine with your dog:

- Mix walking with squats or incorporate sprints into a game of fetch. Aim for at least 30 minutes of continuous aerobic activity daily.
- Engage in your favorite physical activity that elevates your heart rate, adjusting the intensity and duration based on your dog's breed, age, and health.

Moving with your dog—even something as simple as squats—counts toward your daily exercise dose. Take a look at this data summarized from the Centers for Disease Control and Prevention (CDC):[12]

- Only 53.3 percent of adults met the Physical Activity Guidelines for aerobic activity![13]

---

[12] https://www.cdc.gov/nchs/fastats/exercise.htm

[13] Du, Y., et al. "Trends in Adherence to the Physical Activity Guidelines for Americans for Aerobic Activity and Time Spent on Sedentary Behavior Among US Adults, 2007 to 2016." *JAMA Network Open* 2, no. 7 (2019).

- Only 23.2 percent of adults met the Physical Activity Guidelines for both aerobic and muscle-strengthening activity![14]

Aerobic activity involves physical movement that strengthens your heart and lungs by enhancing your body's ability to use oxygen efficiently (aerobic means "with oxygen"). Essentially, any activity that raises your heart rate and breathing qualifies as aerobic activity. As you exert more effort, your body works harder to deliver oxygen to your muscles, causing you to breathe more heavily. I usually recommend starting with a sustained activity for 5–10 minutes, gradually increasing to 10–20 minutes on average. The ultimate goal is to reach 30 minutes of continuous aerobic activity daily—a fantastic target for busy dog owners.

Examples of aerobic activities include brisk walking (my favorite!), jogging, running, biking, swimming, dancing, rowing, playing sports, and any Dog'ercise movements. If an activity raises your heart rate and breathing, it is likely aerobic exercise. We see this in our dogs when they play or run hard and then pause to catch their breath. That is aerobic exercise, and it's great for them as well.

Are we ensuring a daily dose of aerobic exercise for ourselves or our dogs? Look to those around you—look to the left and right. It appears to be an incredibly low percentage, doesn't it? Let's work to raise those numbers and create a healthier life for you and your doggy companion. No, we do not have dog scientists in a lab, collecting data, and researching physical activity to advance

---

[14] Elgaddal, N., and Kramarow, E. A. "Physical Activity Among Adults Aged 65 and Over: United States, 2022." *National Health Statistics Reports* no. 185. Hyattsville, MD: National Center for Health Statistics, 2024.

the well-being of their fellow canines! Instead, we rely on veterinarians and other organizations that provide guidelines for us to follow.

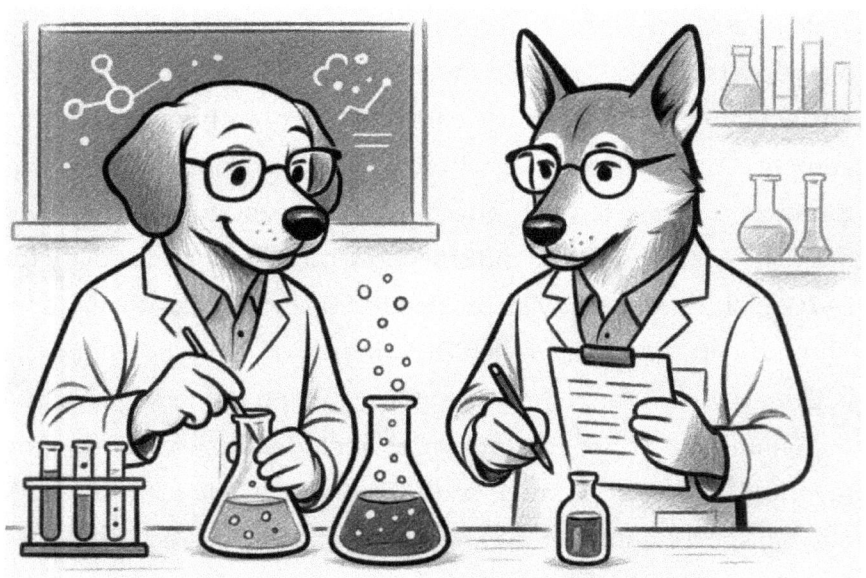

EDUCATIONAL INSIGHTS

- Study your dog's breed characteristics to better understand their exercise needs.
- Adjust activities based on age; puppies and senior dogs have different requirements.
- Consult a veterinarian before starting any new exercise routine.
- Adjust exercise intensity to suit your dog's size and weight.

- Recognize your dog's unique needs and adjust their exercise routines accordingly.
- Vary your dog's activities to keep them engaged and prevent boredom.
- Prioritize regular, consistent exercise over intense, sporadic workouts.
- Monitor for signs of fatigue or discomfort and adjust activities as necessary.

Check out Appendix C for organizations that provide valuable resources for dog owners, including breed information, health and nutrition considerations, and developmental milestones for different breeds.

Remember, the key is to balance physical activity, mental stimulation, and rest, taking into account your dog's unique traits and health needs. Regular checkups with your veterinarian help ensure your choices support your dog's overall well-being.

STORY

Max, a high-energy border collie, exhibited behavioral issues due to insufficient exercise. His owner, Sarah, consulted a vet and discovered the breed's high energy requirements. By adding daily runs and mentally stimulating games to his routine, Max's behavior improved significantly. This story emphasizes the importance of recognizing and fulfilling your dog's exercise needs to support their overall well-being.

Picture yourself as a busy professional, juggling work and personal life. Your energetic Labrador retriever begins showing destructive behavior. Feeling guilty and stressed, you consult your vet, who explains that your dog needs more exercise. Establishing a structured exercise routine improves your dog's behavior and deepens your bond, bringing joy and relief to both of you.

RECOMMENDATIONS

- Evaluate your dog's breed characteristics and energy levels.
- Consult with a veterinarian to design a suitable exercise plan.
- Incorporate a mix of physical and mental activities.
- Monitor your dog's response and adjust activities as needed.
- Establish regular, consistent exercise routines.
- Implement resets in your own and your dog's diet for optimal health.

SUMMARY

Prioritize a balanced lifestyle for you and your dog to ensure a healthy, happy companionship. There's a lot to digest, but researching your dog's breed in advance and having ongoing discussions with your veterinarian are key to understanding the best amount of exercise needed to keep your dog healthy throughout their life. Just a friendly reminder, it's important to select a dog breed and size that matches your typical activity level. This ensures that both you and your dog can safely Dog'ercise together as we explore different age groups. Remember, that is the goal of this book—to help you stay active and pain-free while ensuring your companion can keep up with your activity level. It's a win-win—moving better together just like a hound dog on the trail. *Woof!*

TIP #6
MATCH ACTIVITY LEVELS. ESTABLISH RESETS

CHAPTER 8

PAWS AND FITNESS: A DUAL PATH TO HEALTH AND HAPPINESS

Injury prevention keeps you on your feet and your dog safe on all four paws. Let's explore how you and your dog can stay active and healthy together while reducing potential medical costs.

HUMAN ELEMENT

Staying physically active is essential for maintaining good health as you age. The CDC and the American College of Sports Medicine (ACSM) recommend that adults engage in at least 150 minutes of moderate-intensity aerobic activity each week and incorporate muscle-strengthening activities at least two times each week.[15] However, the ideal amount of exercise depends on your fitness level and pre-existing health conditions.

Before beginning any exercise program, consult your doctor, PT, or a certified healthcare professional. They can help you

---

[15] Garber, Carol E., et al. "Quantity and Quality of Exercise for Developing and Maintaining Cardiorespiratory, Musculoskeletal, and Neuromotor Fitness in Apparently Healthy Adults: Guidance for Prescribing Exercise." *Medicine & Science in Sports & Exercise* 43, no. 7 (2011): 1334-1359.

select safe and appropriate activities for your specific needs. Regular aerobic exercises like walking, swimming, or cycling can significantly improve your cardiovascular health. Strength training, such as weightlifting or resistance band workouts, helps preserve muscle mass and bone density.

Experts recommend including at least 5–10 minutes of stretching into your daily routine. Flexibility and balance exercises like yoga or tai chi help prevent stiffness and reduce the risk of falls.

> Fact: Staying active with your dog can greatly help you meet your recommended physical activity guidelines. First, let's review the general guidelines the CDC and ACSM provided.[16]

HOW MUCH EXERCISE IS THE RIGHT AMOUNT?

That depends on your current fitness level, as well as your dog's age and breed. Do you know how old you are? I most certainly hope so! If not, just count the cracks, pops, and unusual sounds your body makes.

- "Why am I soooo stiff?"—every morning, every evening, anytime you've been sitting for a short period.
- "Does anyone else hear that?"—referring to the loud, unmistakable pops that accompany every joint movement.

---

[16] Garber, "Quantity and Quality," 1334-1359; https://www.cdc.gov/physicalactivity/basics/age-chart.html

- "It takes me about an hour in the morning to get my body's engine moving." Motion is lotion—you just need to grease those joints!
- "Why am I so sore?" or "Where did this bruise come from?"

In summary, when playing fetch with your dog, start slowly. Once you stop moving, it's game over and a slippery slope. The key is to keep the ball in motion. As you age, your throws might not go as far, but as long as you are tossing the ball, you're moving, you're staying active, and so is your dog. Dual movement. Dual lubrication. I hope you WILCO.

DOG CARE

Your dog's age and breed are key factors in determining the right amount of exercise for them. Younger dogs and high-energy breeds require regular activity to burn off excess energy and maintain their health. In contrast, older dogs or those with health issues may benefit from low-impact exercises to protect their joints and prevent strains.

Like humans, dogs benefit from both aerobic and strength training exercises. Activities like fetching, running, and agility training help keep them physically fit. For older dogs, swimming or gentle walks are excellent ways to keep them active without putting excessive strain on their joints.

It is important to monitor your dog's response to exercise. If they show signs of fatigue, discomfort, or pain, stop the activity and consult your veterinarian. Keeping your dog hydrated and providing a balanced diet is essential for maintaining their overall health and energy levels.

SAMPLE WORKOUTS

- Start with a brisk 5-minute walk as a warm-up. Incorporate a variety of activities below to stay active—I recommend mixing up your routine each week. I call this "building the armor" to prepare your body for everyday stressors like lifting a heavy box, installing a ceiling fan, changing a tire, or tackling household or yard tasks. End with a 5-minute cooldown walk and some gentle stretching.
- Incorporate Aerobic Exercise: Engage in regular aerobic activities such as walking, swimming, cycling, or low-impact aerobics. Aim for at least 30 minutes of moderately intense aerobic exercise five times a week. An example of moderate intensity is brisk walking, where you breathe heavily and can still talk but can't sing. If you use a scaling system where zero would be easy and 10 would be the most difficult, you should be in the 5–6 range.
- Include Strength Training: Incorporate strength training exercises to maintain muscle mass and bone density. Focus on major muscle groups with activities like weightlifting, resistance band exercises, or bodyweight workouts. Include strength training at least two times a week.
- Prioritize Flexibility and Balance: Include flexibility exercises to maintain joint mobility and prevent stiffness. I recommend 5–10 minutes of daily stretching to support your body as we

age. Yoga, Pilates, and tai chi are excellent for enhancing flexibility, improving balance, and reducing the risk of falls.
- Choose Low-Impact Activities: Opt for low-impact exercises to reduce stress on joints. Activities like swimming, elliptical training, and stationary cycling provide a great workout while being gentler on the joints.
- Stay Active Throughout the Day: Integrate movement into your daily routine by taking short walks, opting for stairs over elevators, or incorporating simple exercises during breaks.
- Listen to Your Body: Listen to your body's response to exercise. If you experience pain, shortness of breath, dizziness, or any unusual symptoms, stop immediately and consult your healthcare provider. Remember, "no pain, no gain" does NOT apply. Pushing through discomfort can lead to injury.
- Include Social Activities: Participate in group workouts or activities to make exercise more enjoyable and stay motivated. Socializing with others enhances the experience, whether you're moving with friends, family, or your dog, because moving better together makes adventures more fun!
- Modify Exercises Accordingly: Don't hesitate to modify exercises if you're in a class or if something feels off. Pushing through discomfort can lead to injury. Adapt exercises to match your fitness level and any physical limitations. Adjust the intensity, duration, or activity to ensure a safe and effective workout.
- Hydrate and Fuel Properly: Stay hydrated and maintain a balanced diet to support your energy and overall well-being.

Proper nutrition is crucial for maintaining muscle strength, bone health, and sustained physical activity.
- Get Regular Checkups: Regular health checkups become increasingly important as you age. They help detect and address any potential health concerns early, allowing you to make the necessary adjustments to your exercise routine.

EDUCATIONAL INSIGHTS

- Understand your dog's age and breed-specific exercise requirements.
- Schedule regular vet checkups to monitor your dog's health and adjust their exercise routine accordingly.
- Always provide fresh water before, during, and after exercise to keep them hydrated.
- Be mindful of weather conditions—avoid intense activities in extreme heat or cold.

STORY

Remy, an 8-year-old Labrador retriever, had become increasingly sluggish and gained weight over the years. His owner, Karen, knew it was time for a change. They started with short daily walks, gradually increasing the distance, and adding play sessions. Over time, Remy lost weight, regained his energy, and Karen also felt healthier and happier. Their daily exercise routine also strengthened their bond.

Imagine a retired couple, Jane and Robert, who adopted a senior dog named Tucker. Jane struggled with arthritis, and Robert was recovering from a minor heart attack. By adding gentle walks and swimming sessions with Tucker to their daily routine, they improved their physical health and also found joy and companionship. Their bond with Tucker gave them a renewed sense of purpose and happiness in their golden years.

RECOMMENDATIONS

- Consult your doctor and vet before starting a new exercise program.
- Include aerobic, strength, and flexibility exercises in your routine.
- Choose low-impact exercises to protect your joints.
- Stay active throughout the day with small, manageable activities.
- Keep yourself and your dog hydrated and maintain a balanced diet.
- Schedule regular checkups for both you and your dog.

SUMMARY

Staying active with your dog not only improves your health but also deepens your bond. It's never too late to start a new routine that benefits both you and your furry companion. Exercising with your dog helps you meet recommended physical activity guidelines while maintaining overall health and functionality. The key is to find activities you enjoy, making exercise more enjoyable and sustainable. Take it slow and steady; it's the best approach for you and your dog.

TIP #7
KNOW YOUR AGE. STAY INJURY-FREE.

CHAPTER 9

CORE ESSENTIALS: STRENGTHENING HEALTH FOR HUMANS AND DOGS

A strong core is essential for preventing injuries and maintaining overall health and fitness, not just for humans, but for our canine companions. Injury prevention reduces healthcare costs, minimizes the need for medical treatment, and enhances quality of life. By incorporating regular exercise and a core-strengthening routine, both you and our dog stay healthy, active, and happy.

HUMAN ELEMENT

Following guidelines from the CDC and ACSM can help ensure you get the right amount and type of physical activity. The core of your body, which includes the gluteus maximus, hips, abdominal muscles, diaphragm, pelvic floor muscles, and paraspinal muscles, plays a crucial role in stabilizing your body and enabling efficient movement. Strengthening these muscles helps prevent injuries and improve overall functionality. This is especially important for those who have experienced back pain, a condition that affects over 80 percent of people at some point in their lives.[17]

To evaluate your core strength, try these simple tests:

- Squat Test: Hold a low squat position for as long as possible—hips down, chest up. This measures the strength and endurance of your core muscles.
- Plank test: Make a straight line with your body and hold a plank on your elbows to see how long you can maintain it. How long can you last? Try to gradually increase your time.

As you work to improve your physical activity and overall health, it's important to acknowledge your age and limitations. Each decade brings about its own unique challenges and changes as your body experiences natural wear and tear. Embrace the joys, tackle the challenges, and find ways to enjoy every stage of life. Remember, you are the captain of your journey, and the sails are yours to control. The key is being aware of your age and adapting accordingly.

You might not feel your actual biological age and might even feel much younger. Some adults tell me they never truly "grew up" and still feel like they're stuck in their twenties. I can relate; I often feel like I am in my twenties on most days. Other days? Not so much. Some people, however, may feel (or even look) like Barney Rubble—maybe a bit like Dino. You know, the ones who make you do a double take. *Ruff!* All these factors are shaped by your lifestyle choices over the years.

---

[17] Hoy, Douglas, et al. "A Systematic Review of the Global Prevalence of Low Back Pain." *Arthritis & Rheumatism* 64, no. 6 (2012): 2028-2037.

Of course, genetics plays a role, but your lifestyle has the power to either slow down or accelerate, or speed up the genetic factors you are predisposed to. I'm no geneticist, but I know healthy habits—like eating well, getting enough sleep (not my favorite, but definitely my wife's), and regular exercise are key ingredients for well-being! Other essential ingredients? Laughter and fun! Ultimately, you create your own recipe for a healthy, fulfilling life.

This book focuses on another key ingredient—exercise—along with a few laughs. Call it a *CORE* workout. Just laugh harder, and you will feel it in your abdominal muscles. The best (or worst) part? When these muscles are very sore, and then you start laughing or sneezing; I'm never sure whether to cry or yell on those days.

While we're on this topic—THE CORE—let's define what that actually means. And no, it doesn't need to be capitalized; it looks more dramatic. The word *core* is not a mysterious made-up term; it has multiple meanings. Think of the core of an apple, the earth's core, an organization's core values, or your core values. Are you blown away yet? It's a pretty cool word to describe the central or most important part of something. One of my favorite definitions came from a patient I worked with many years ago—a flight attendant. I was explaining what the core is, and our conversation went like this:

Patient (let's call her Ms. Awesome, because she truly was): "You mean the core is like a fuselage?"

Me: "Huh?"

Ms. Awesome: "The fuselage."

Me: "Is that French?"

Ms. Awesome: "Um, possibly. In aeronautics, it's the main body of the aircraft where passengers or cargo sit."

Me: "Yes! That is exactly how you can think of the core of the body. How do you spell that again?"

I had to look it up later—it turns out fuselage sounds like one bad mama jama. In other words, the *core*!

Think of your core as your body's fuselage (go ahead, look it up). Its muscles work together to provide stability to your center—your trunk—so your arms and legs can move efficiently. Did you ever do the Y.M.C.A. dance, spelling out the letters Y–M–C–A with your arms? You need a strong core just to lift your arms above your head.

Just like an aircraft needs its fuselage to support the wings and tail, your body relies on its core for stability and movement. You wouldn't go far with just the wings or the tail—the fuselage holds everything together. Let that sink in on your next layover while you're doing squats, lunges, and planks in the terminal.

And just because you can wave your arms around like it's no big deal doesn't necessarily mean you have a strong core. Just saying. *Ruff! Ugh.*

DOG CARE

Just like humans, dogs greatly benefit from a strong core. Their core muscles, especially those along the spine, play a crucial role in maintaining stability and supporting movements like sitting, standing, and transitioning between positions. This is particularly important for dogs with longer backs or breeds prone to spinal issues. Strengthening your dog's core can help prevent injuries, enhance mobility, and improve overall quality of life.

SAMPLE WORKOUTS

Incorporate Dog'ercise into other activities:

- Fetch and Sprint: Throw a ball or toy, then walk backward, sprint, or side-shuffle alongside your dog to retrieve it.
- Obstacle Course: Create a mini obstacle course with hurdles, tunnels, and weave poles to navigate with your dog.
- Tug-of-War: This strengthens your dog's core while providing you with a good upper body workout.

What do we physical therapists look for in a strong core? It is not just about muscle strength but also how well those muscles work together to support your body. Physical therapists evaluate both the strength and coordination of the core muscles described earlier.

Here are some simple clinical tests to help you evaluate your core strength. Try them out to determine your core baseline.

SQUATS

How long can you maintain a moderately deep squat without going all the way down to your heels?

HEALTHY LIVING WITH YOUR DOG

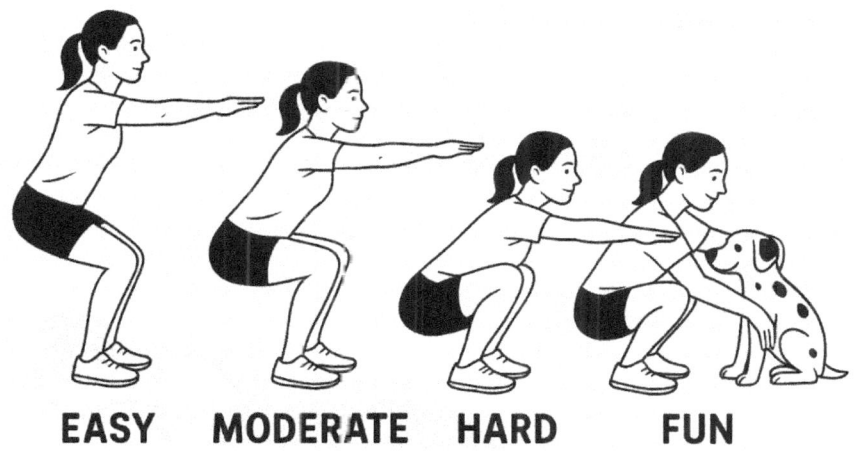

How low can you go?

SCORE	TIME	COMMENTS
Less than 15 seconds	_____	Let's step it up, trooper!
16–30 seconds	_____	A bit more effort to strengthen your baseline.
31–45 seconds	_____	About where you should be, at the minimum.
46–60 seconds	_____	Great job, partner!
Over 60 seconds	_____	You have a strong set of armor—well done!

FRONT AND SIDE PLANKS

Use the same scoring to assess your progress with the following exercises. Keep track of your baseline to monitor improvement over time.

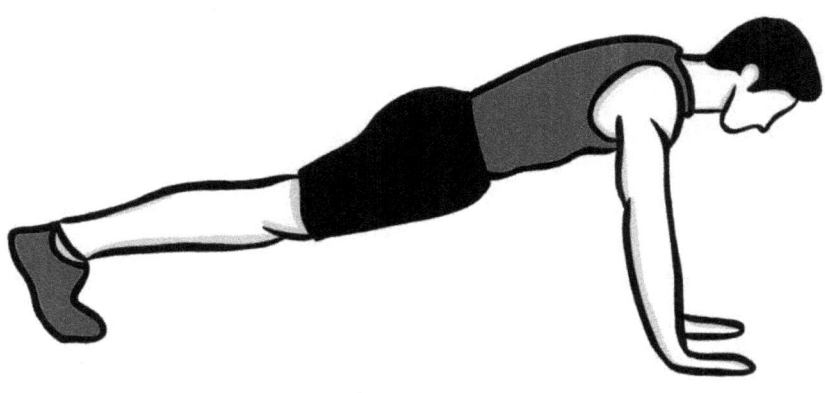

Front plank

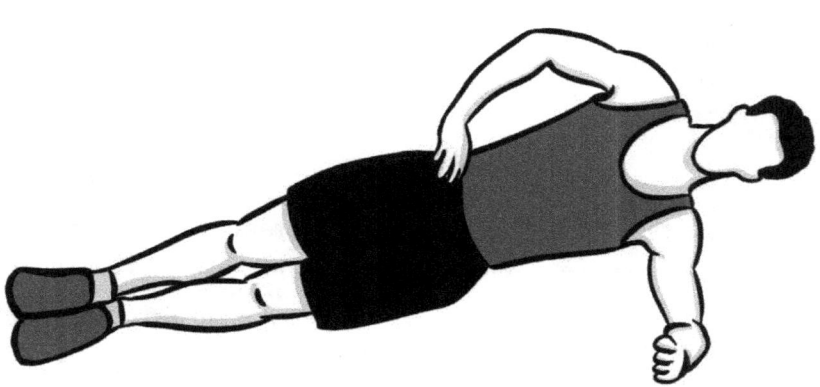

Side plank

BRIDGES:

Can you hold a bridge for one minute?

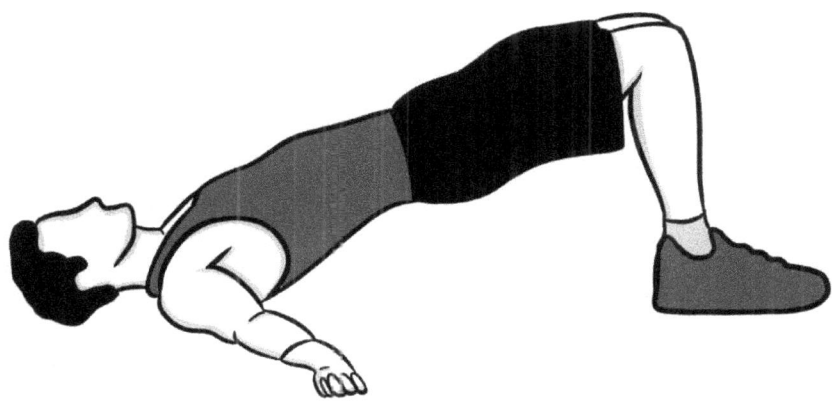

Bridge

What about a single-leg bridge on each leg?

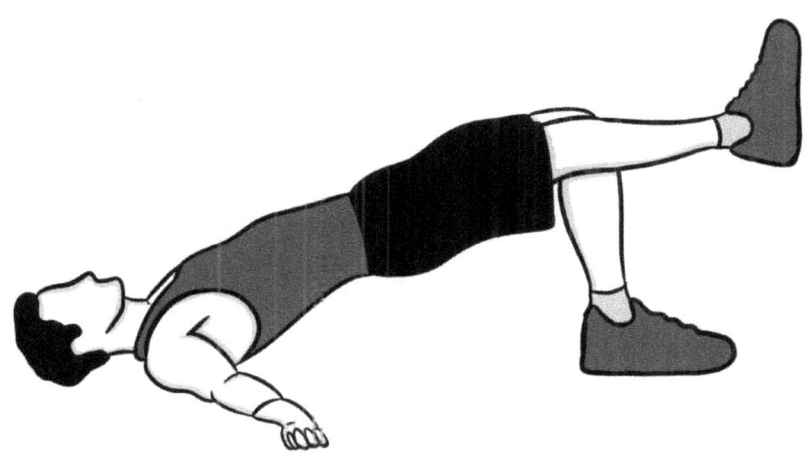

Single-legged bridge

How long can you maintain balance on each leg?
Baseline:

        Right Foot   seconds

        Left Foot   seconds

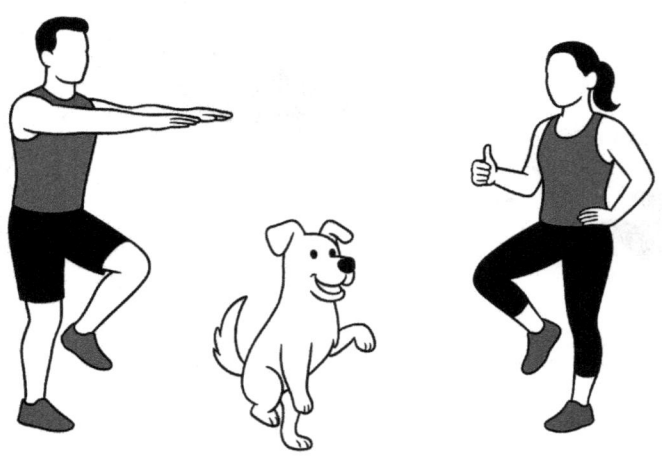

Balancing is fun!

Periodically retest throughout the year to monitor your progress and identify any setbacks if your routine has been inconsistent.

If any of these exercises sound unfamiliar, consult your PT or trainer.

These simple tests help determine if your body has a stable fuselage. These exercises can assess your core strength like an auto mechanic diagnosing your car.

Truthfully, there isn't a standardized core strength test for dogs. However, if they can roll over, stand on their hind legs, and move comfortably, it's a safe bet their fuselages are engaged. Unlike humans, dogs don't spend hours watching TV or scrolling through social media, so they don't develop sedentary habits as long as they're exercised.

Dogs have a naturally low center of gravity, and strong core muscles are essential for supporting their spine and preventing injuries. This is especially important for dogs with longer backs or breeds prone to spinal issues. They rely on their core for everyday movements like sitting, standing, and transitioning between positions. Since these actions are part of their daily routine, they naturally have a strong core.

TIP #8
BUILD A STRONG CORE.
FORTIFY YOUR FOUNDATION.

EDUCATIONAL INSIGHTS

- A strong core is essential for preventing injuries and maintaining overall health and fitness.
- Optimizing core muscle activation is essential for joint protection, spinal support, and maintaining quality of life for humans and dogs.

STORY

Let's revisit one of my favorite stories about Ms. Awesome, a flight attendant who compared the body's core to the fuselage of an aircraft. This analogy perfectly illustrates the core's role as the central structure that provides support and stability, just like the fuselage holds together an aircraft's wings and tail. Her clever comparison made the concept of core strength both relatable and memorable.

Imagine a middle-aged individual who has been inactive for years and starts experiencing lower back pain. Determined to make a change, they begin a structured exercise program focusing on core strength. Over time, they notice significant improvements in mobility and a reduction in pain. This story highlights the power of core training in transforming lives, reducing pain, and increasing overall well-being.

RECOMMENDATIONS

For Humans:
- Follow the CDC and ACSM guidelines for physical activity.
- Incorporate core-strengthening exercises into your routine.
- Regularly assess your core strength using the simple tests outlined in this chapter.

For Dogs:
- Engage in activities that strengthen your dog's core.
- Monitor your dog's mobility and adjust exercises as needed.
- Maintain their healthy weight to minimize stress on their spine.

SUMMARY

As we work toward increasing physical activity and improving our health, it's essential to understand our age and physical limits. Embrace each stage of life, cherish the joys, and find fun in every moment. Remember, you are the captain of your ship, and only you can steer the course. Prioritizing core strength for you and your furry friend helps prevent injuries and enhances overall well-being.

The core of the body is like the fuselage of an aircraft, providing stability and strength for every movement.
—Ms. Awesome

CHAPTER 10

PROACTIVE HEALTH FOR YOU AND YOUR DOG: ENJOY ADVENTURES

Caring for both your body and your dog's means taking proactive steps to ensure many years of adventures together. Injury prevention is key; it keeps you both active and helps reduce medical costs by minimizing the need for treatments and interventions.

Now, let's explore how understanding the connection between human and canine age, managing portion sizes, and taking preventive measures can help you and your dog continue enjoying life's adventures.

HUMAN ELEMENT

UNDERSTANDING HUMAN AGE AND HEALTH

Understanding how age affects our bodies is crucial for maintaining health and preventing injuries. A common myth suggests that one human year equals seven dog years; however, research indicates that aging is more complex. Advances in healthcare have increased life expectancy, and a deeper understanding of how the human body changes over time can help individuals maintain their health for longer periods.

THE IMPORTANCE OF PORTION CONTROL

Portion control is crucial for maintaining a healthy weight and reducing the risk of disease. Excess food is stored as fat, often in areas that put extra strain on vital organs. Proper portion management ensures we provide our bodies with the right amount of fuel for energy without unnecessary fat storage.

THE ROLE OF PHYSICAL THERAPY

Regular checkups with a PT or other healthcare provider can help maintain optimal body movement and function. A PT tune-up includes evaluating joints, strength, and range of motion to prevent injuries and promote healthy movement patterns. Most states in the USA have direct access to PTs, allowing you to receive expert care without a referral. I may be biased as a physical therapist, but I firmly believe everyone should have an annual physical therapy checkup, just like a routine exam with their physician.

The same principle applies to your canine friend and their routine veterinary exams. The PT tune-up provides a full-body assessment, starting with the all-mighty core and then evaluating joints, strength, and range of motion—a complete "tune-up" for your body. Think of it like taking your car to a mechanic. You wouldn't want them to check just one issue—you'd expect a full inspection to catch any potential problems. You should take the same approach with your health.

DOG CARE

CALCULATING DOG YEARS

The old belief that one human year equals seven dog years is outdated. Modern research, including insights from the American Kennel Club (AKC), shows that a dog's aging process is more complex and influenced by factors like breed, size, and genetics. Understanding your dog's true age helps ensure they receive the proper care for their specific needs.

WEIGHT MANAGEMENT FOR DOGS

Maintaining your dog's healthy weight is crucial for their overall well-being. Excess weight increases the risk of various health issues as they age. Proper portion control and regular exercise are key to maintaining a healthy weight and ensuring a longer, happier life for your dog.

REGULAR VET CHECKUPS

Just as humans benefit from regular checkups with a PT, dogs need routine exams with a veterinarian. These checkups can help detect health issues early and ensure your dog remains in good health. Being proactive about your dog's healthcare can prevent more serious problems in the future.

Before we explore the comparison of human age to canine age, I would like to acknowledge the AKC for their valuable insights on "How to Calculate Dog Years to Human Years." For more in-depth information, visit their website: https://www.akc.org.

The notion that one human year equals seven dog years is a long-standing myth. While this rule has been around since the mid-1950s, based on an average human life of seventy years and a dog's lifespan of ten years, it no longer holds true.

Advances in technology, healthcare, and scientific understanding have increased life expectancy for humans and dogs. According to the AKC and a 2019 study a more accurate method for estimating a dog's age is by examining changes in its DNA over time. As we've discussed, the aging process varies widely among different breeds and sizes of dogs, making a one-size-fits-all formula unrealistic.

It makes sense that a dog's size, traits, activity levels, and genetics all contribute to determining its equivalent human age. Since the research in this area is still evolving, experts hypothesize that excess weight in dogs may increase the risk of diseases as they age. This emphasizes the importance of proper weight management in supporting healthy aging in our canine companions.

Our therapy clinic uses a fancy machine that measures visceral adipose tissue—a.k.a the 'bad fat." This unhealthy fat accumulates deep in the abdominal cavity surrounding vital organs, from your neck to midline. This lard, blub, the extra-thick stuff—you know what I'm talking about. This fat can put added pressure on your internal organs, increasing health risks even though it's not visible outside your body.

This is why portion control is crucial when fueling yourself and your dog with food. Excess fuel is stored as fat throughout our bodies—often in less-than-ideal areas, like the abdomen, chin, or thighs. If only we could choose where to store extra fat, we'd eat everything in sight.

We're all wired a bit differently when it comes to our relationship with food. If you eat a large meal, that's totally fine—I do it all the time because, well, food is heavenly. However, when I do, I often skip my next meal, allowing my body to use that fuel efficiently. I'm not worried about starving; I know food is always available when I need it. My wife, on the other hand, has a different approach. Skipping a meal would make her "hangry" in no time—and trust me, neither of us wants that!

If you stop and think about it, food is all around us! The key is figuring out how your body responds to it. I prefer to burn off my meals if I decide to indulge in a big one. So, ask yourself—are you a *storer* or a *burner*?

To help your body to store fuel, keep eating large meals daily. Just remember—your choices don't just affect you, but also impact your dog's health. Be mindful of their nutrition just as you are with your own.

I'll doggone bet you that carrying extra junk in the trunk will come back to bite you—mostly in a bad way. Fat itself isn't the enemy; in fact, it is a valuable source of energy. Let me repeat that—fat is *good* when consumed in *moderation*. Our brains thrive on fat for energy, but excessive fat intake can lead to unhealthy cholesterol levels (LDL, VLDL), which negatively impact your heart and arteries. Heart attacks and strokes—oh my! Let's avoid these, people. You can't keep on living if you're in the ground. RIP.

I hate to be the bearer of bad news, but let's set the record straight. If you are taller, yes, you'll have longer bones. However, if your excuse is, "I'm just big-boned," you're barking up the wrong tree and off track for Tip #2. *Don't do that.* Some research suggests that carrying a little extra weight can help you live longer, and I won't argue or bark with that. Having a bit of extra storage is fine, but *obesity*? Bad dog—bad!

Imagine your vital organs inside your fuselage getting suffocated by excess fat. That's when it's time to call in the special forces to take out the bad guys. While you may not have access to Delta Force—the elite combat unit trained for special operations—you *do* have your dog. And together, you can go on the attack, one activity at a time.

It's all about movement, my friends. Become a fuel burner. Over time, consistent activity will help improve weight management and eliminate excess fat—especially the unhealthy stuff.

Guess what? The more muscle you build and the more active you are, the more fuel you burn. This means you can eat more food! If you love food, move more.

Got it? Say no more. That's the spirit!

SAMPLE WORKOUTS

Check the calendar and choose one day each week for a new and exciting adventure, e.g., a trail to explore or a lake for swimming. It could even be a new dog park to explore and meet some new friends.

EDUCATIONAL INSIGHTS

- Regular Checkups: Schedule regular health exams for both you and your dog.

- Portion Control: Maintain a healthy weight by managing portion sizes.
- Exercise Together: Engage in regular physical activities with your dog.
- Stay Informed: Keep up with the latest research and guidelines on health and fitness for both you and your dog.

STORY

Imagine a dog named Luna and her owner, Sarah. When Sarah noticed Luna gaining weight and slowing down, she took her to the vet and learned that she was at risk for diabetes. Determined to help Luna, she introduced a new routine that included daily walks, portion control, and regular vet checkups. Over time, Luna lost weight, regained her energy, and their bond grew even stronger. This story highlights the importance of taking proactive steps to protect both your and your dog's well-being.

Picture this: You're hiking on a beautiful trail with your dog when they suddenly start limping. An old injury has flared up, and you realize that this could have been prevented with more regular vet checkups and exercise. This emotional moment emphasizes the importance of preventive care and staying active, ensuring both you and your dog can enjoy life's adventures without setbacks.

RECOMMENDATIONS

- Schedule Annual Checkups: Visit your physician, PT, or other healthcare provider.

- Prioritize Vet Visits: Ensure your dog receives routine veterinary checkups to monitor their health.
- Practice Portion Control: Maintain a balanced diet for both you and your dog to achieve a healthy weight.
- Commit to Regular Exercise: Establish consistent physical activity routines for both you and your furry companion.
- Stay Educated: Keep up with the latest health and fitness guidelines to make informed decisions for you and your dog.

SUMMARY

A proactive approach to your and your dog's health leads to a longer, happier life filled with adventures. Small, consistent steps, such as regular checkups, exercise, and proper nutrition, can help prevent injuries and illnesses, allowing for quality time together.

In summary, the annual medical checkup is essential for assessing your *inner core*—including blood work, cholesterol levels, heart function, and lung health. However, a tune-up with your PT to evaluate your *musculoskeletal core*—strength, range of motion, balance, and coordination—ensures your body moves safely and efficiently.

This proactive approach naturally leads to a healthier, more active lifestyle with a lower risk of injury and less pain! *Kaboom!*

Quality movement helps prevent compensation and reduces the risk of additional pain. Most states in the US offer direct access to physical therapy, allowing you to see a PT without a doctor's referral. Check with your insurance provider or consider paying out of pocket—cash payments can sometimes be more affordable.

Direct access allows you to receive care from a PT more quickly, saving time and reducing healthcare costs. Finally, something the healthcare system got right!

TIP #9
BE PROACTIVE. STAY TUNED UP.

CHAPTER 11

ACTIVE LIVES, HAPPY LIVES: INJURY PREVENTION AND FITNESS FOR KIDS AND DOGS

Injury prevention is important at any age and plays a vital role in maintaining a healthy lifestyle while reducing medical expenses. Staying physically active helps prevent injuries and supports overall well-being.

By adopting fun and regular exercise routines, both you and your dog remain fit and healthy. Let's take a look at where it all begins—from duckling to flight, from crawling to running—here we go!

Kids thrive when they move and have fun, so focus on activities that develop speed, coordination, and balance. Similarly, dogs benefit from early training with positive reinforcement. A consistent routine is key to success for both humans and dogs

HUMAN ELEMENT

Preschool-Aged Children (3–5 years): Let kids be kids! Encourage them to explore, ask questions, and learn through movement. Ensure they spend plenty of time outdoors engaging in physical activities they enjoy. At this stage, both mental and physical strength are developing, making it an ideal time to focus on speed, coordination, balance, and reaction drills.

Activities like playing catch, sprinting, and climbing help train the nervous system and improve movement quality. Speed, quickness, and agility are what set top athletes apart from the rest.

Engage in activities with your kids, showing them that exercise can be enjoyable while also meeting your daily physical activity goals. This keeps them active, reduces screen time, and strengthens your bond—a perfect trifecta.

Exposing children to a variety of sports and activities helps develop overall athleticism by challenging different muscle groups and movement patterns. While genetics plays a role, maximizing potential through diverse experiences is key. Plus, the more active the kids are, the faster they will fall asleep at night, giving you some well-deserved time for yourself.

Including your dog in family playtime helps them become well-integrated members of the family. Early exposure to kids can be beneficial, but seek expert advice to ensure a smooth and safe introduction.

Encourage breaks and establish healthy snack routines after physical activities. Starting early helps children reach their full potential and instills valuable life skills for the future.

DOG CARE

Puppy Stage (less than one year): This stage is all about play, support, fun, and nurturing. Short walks, obedience training, and plenty of sleep are essential for their growth and development.

Puppies will let you know when they're tired—usually by plopping down on the spot. At this stage, focus on creating lots of laughs and minimizing stress to help your pup develop into a happy, well-adjusted companion.

Stay calm and positive when accidents happen—like a knocked-over garbage can. Use these moments as opportunities to teach responsibility and ownership. Get the whole family involved in the cleanup to turn a chore into a fun, interactive experience. Life is short, especially for dogs, so make the most of every day.

Exercise your puppy in short, frequent sessions, gradually increasing the duration as they grow. Consistency is key—finding a fun and safe routine will set you and your dog up for long-term success.

As Dwayne Johnson wisely said, "Success isn't always about greatness. It's about consistency. Consistent hard work leads to success. Greatness will come."

SAMPLE WORKOUTS

Incorporate a variety of fun and engaging activities that you and your dog can enjoy together. Start with age-appropriate toys to provide mental and physical stimulation. Sometimes, simply getting on the floor during a cooldown session with some light stretching is enough to spark laughter and playful puppy licks.

EDUCATIONAL INSIGHTS

- Start Early: Use age-appropriate exercises and begin training and socializing your dog at a young age.

- Mix It Up: Introduce a variety of activities to keep your dog mentally and physically engaged.
- Stay Consistent: Maintain a regular exercise routine to build healthy habits.
- Reward Good Behavior: Use treats and praise to reinforce positive actions.
- Prioritize Hydration and Rest: Make sure your dog stays hydrated and gets sufficient rest after exercise.

STORY

Once upon a time, a family adopted a playful puppy named Shadow. Shadow loved running around the yard, playing fetch, and going on walks with his new family. One day, however, Shadow got into the trash and made a mess. Instead of scolding him, the family laughed it off, turned the cleanup into a game, and made it a fun experience for everyone, including Shadow. This story reminds us of the power of patience, positive reinforcement, and finding joy in everyday moments.

Imagine a child and a dog growing up together, staying active, and learning healthy habits. The child develops excellent coordination and athletic skills, while the dog becomes a fit, well-behaved companion. Their bond fosters a passion for movement, cultivating lifelong habits that enhance overall well-being and reduce the risk of injuries.

RECOMMENDATIONS

- Make Movement a Daily Habit: Engage in regular physical activities with your children and dog.
- Keep It Fun and Engaging: Incorporate a variety of exercises to keep workouts interesting and challenging.
- Encourage with Positivity: Use treats, praise, and play to reinforce good behavior in your dog.
- Prioritize Health and Safety: Regularly monitor both your child and dog for signs of fatigue or injury.
- Stay Consistent: Maintain a routine to build lasting healthy habits.

SUMMARY

Encourage your kids and your dog to embrace an active lifestyle—it's one of the greatest gifts you can give them.

TIP #10
ACTIVE LIVES ARE HAPPY LIVES. HAVE FUN!

Opportunity is missed by most people because it is dressed in overalls and looks like work.
—Thomas Edison

CHAPTER 12

HEALTHY AND ACTIVE TOGETHER: EXERCISE AND INJURY PREVENTION

Proper exercise form is crucial for long-term health and significantly reduces the risk of injuries. By using correct techniques and following exercise guidelines for both humans and dogs, you can enjoy an active lifestyle while minimizing the risk of injuries. This proactive approach not only reduces medical costs but also enhances overall well-being.

HUMAN ELEMENT

CHILDREN AND ADOLESCENTS

Growing up is so much fun! For children ages 6–17 years, aim for at least 60 minutes of moderate to vigorous physical activity each day. This supports physical development—improving strength, balance, coordination, and athleticism—and enhances mental agility.

Team sports, such as soccer, hockey, and basketball are excellent for developing essential life skills, including work ethic, communication, teamwork, and motivation. Kids also learn listening skills and the importance of self-sacrifice. Even professional athletes emphasize that success often comes from making sacrifices to reach their goals. I once treated a National Football League player who shared a valuable lesson about sacrifice. He explained that staying focused on his goals and making intentional sacrifices, like skipping parties and limiting TV time, helped him reach the elite level in his sport. This lesson isn't just for professional athletes; it applies to everyone, including kids on their own sports and fitness journeys.

MUSCLE-STRENGTHENING ACTIVITIES

Include muscle-strengthening activities at least three times a week. Exercises like push-ups, crab walks, inchworms, jumping rope, and squats are excellent examples.

To ensure safety and effectiveness:

- Provide proper supervision and guidance.
- Focus on age-appropriate programs with the correct technique.
- Gradually increase resistance and intensity as strength improves.
- Experts highly recommend bodyweight exercises for younger children to build a solid foundation for strength and movement.

To help prevent injuries, emphasize the importance of a strong core, especially for high schoolers who may be lifting heavy weights without proper guidance. Developing good habits and maintaining core strength can help reduce the risk of back pain and other injuries. Encourage proper technique and pay close attention to any signs of pain or discomfort. Seeking professional guidance early can prevent minor issues from becoming chronic ones.

For this age group, aim for at least 60 minutes of moderate to vigorous physical activity daily. A good indicator of intensity is heavier breathing, which makes it clear they're working harder.

As parents, we know that physical activity helps "wear out" our kids, but it also plays a crucial role in developing and maintaining mental agility, athleticism, balance, coordination, and overall muscle engagement.

STRENGTH TRAINING

I don't know about you, but protecting my joints and back is a priority at any age. Like many, I didn't think of this early on and lifted without proper guidance. In my profession, I see firsthand that while weights are beneficial, excessive loads often lead to injuries, regardless of age. I see it all the time in my high school athletes, and it often results in back pain—not good.

That's why Tip #8 is crucial: Build your foundation with a strong core. I cannot stress enough how important this is for long-term success. Trust me, no one reading this wants to be limping, in pain, or facing multiple surgeries down the road. No doggone way!

You do you, but be disciplined and intentional in your approach. If you choose to lift heavy weights, proceed gradually, listen to your body, and avoid overcompensating, as poor form often leads to injury. Start good habits early—focus on athleticism and team sports while you're young. Whatever activities you choose to enjoy with your kids, have fun and stay active, but always prioritize safety.

> **IMPORTANT TIP**
> If the movement looks or feels "off," it probably is—trust your instincts.

What I mean is that if a movement does not look or feel athletic or fluid, it probably isn't. You have likely seen a child or even an adult move in such a way that makes you do a double take. While poor movement patterns can be hard to correct in adulthood, identifying and addressing them early can make a significant difference.

This is the perfect stage to focus on quality movement with the help of a licensed physical therapist (PT), an advanced strength and conditioning coach, or a knowledgeable personal trainer. Learn to move well!

This is also a great time to discuss OPTEMPO—your operational tempo. This refers to maintaining a sustainable rhythm for daily, weekly, or long-term activities, whether in sports or other movement activities. Create a schedule that works for you.

DOG CARE

As dogs grow and mature, they can handle longer distances and more strenuous activities. To prevent injuries, start slowly and gradually increase exercise duration and intensity of exercises. A helpful guideline is the 10 percent rule, which suggests increasing activity levels incrementally to ensure safe progression for anyone increasing activity levels. This helps in increasing mileage, intensity level, or duration of an activity by no more than a 10 percent increase per week for injury prevention. This allows a safe ramp-up to build stronger bones and tissues while adapting to new challenges.

Pay attention to your dog's pace and duration, adjusting them as needed. Running, playing, and varied movements help develop your dog's overall strength and prevent imbalances.

Wolff's Law states that bones adapt to the stress placed on them. Gradually increasing activity levels helps strengthen bones and reduce the risk of injuries, such as shin splints or stress fractures. The same principle applies to dogs, especially those involved in high-impact activities, such as running.

STRENGTH TRAINING FOR DOGS

Just like humans, dogs benefit from strength training. Activities involving varied movements on different terrains, including hills, helps build strength and improve overall fitness. Incorporate these exercises into your dog's routine to promote balanced muscle development and maintain their strength and overall health.

SAMPLE WORKOUTS

A simple workout could include a brisk 10-minute walk with your dog, going up and down hills. Follow this with 10 squats and 10 lunges on hills, then repeat the cycle as often as possible.

To progress safely, gradually increase the duration, intensity, and number of repetitions using the 10 percent rule. This allows both you and your dog to adapt safely to increased physical activity while building strength and endurance.

EDUCATIONAL INSIGHTS

- Begin gradually and increase exercise intensity slowly to prevent injuries.
- Observe your dog's physical condition and adjust activities as needed.
- Incorporate a variety of movements to promote balanced muscle development.
- Consult your veterinarian for personalized exercise recommendations tailored to your dog's needs.

> FACTS: On average, walking a mile is about 2,000 steps, depending on your stride. Research suggests that walking at a faster pace may help you live longer compared to slower walkers—that is great news! I learned to walk quickly just to stay on time for my patients, and now it's a habit. Yippee!

To increase longevity, studies have shown that faster walking speeds are linked to lower mortality rates and a longer life expectancy. [18]

---

[18] Zaccardi, Francesco, et al. "Association of Walking Pace and Handgrip Strength With All-Cause, Cardiovascular, and Cancer Mortality: A UK Biobank Observational Study." *Mayo Clinic Proceedings* 94, no. 4 (2019): 577-588; Celis-Morales, Carlo A., et al. "Self-Reported Walking Pace: A Simple Screening Tool With Lowest Risk of All-Cause Mortality in High-Active Brisk Walkers." *Journal of Sports Sciences* 41, no. 10 (2023): 1068–77.

Other key indicators of longevity include:

- Strong grip
- Good balance
- Ability to get down and up from the floor
- Sitting and standing from a chair without using your hands

Want to learn more? Visit www.movebettertogether.com for more information.

> TEN PERCENT RULE REMINDER: The 10 percent rule recommends increasing exercise duration or intensity by no more than 10 percent each week. This gradual progression helps your body adapt safely to increased activity, minimizing the risk of injury and overtraining.

Listen to your body. Continue until you find the right distance or time that works for you and your dog—when you're both feeling like superstars! Feel free to incorporate additional strengthening exercises as you want within the time have.

> FOR EXPERIENCED FITNESS ENTHUSIASTS: Remember, your young dog is still growing. While you may be ready for long-distance runs, your pup's joints are still developing. Protect their joints by following the 10 percent rule and gradually increasing their activity levels.

For those of you with sporting breeds or dogs built for endurance, ensure your exercise routine includes more than just running.

Running primarily strengthens movement in the sagittal plane, a fancy phrase for forward and backward motion.

Just like the rest of us humans, if runners only run, they can develop weakness in their hip stabilizers and neglect upper body and core strength. As a physical therapist, I frequently encounter runners with knee, hip, or back pain stemming from these imbalances. So, instead of "Run, Forrest, run!" let's change it to "Run, Forrest, fun!" because variety is the key!

The same applies to dogs—if they only run with you and don't engage in play and multidirectional movement, they risk developing muscle imbalances. To build full-body strength, dogs need time to run, jump, and move in various directions a.k.a. playtime! So, strengthening beyond running is key whether it's you or your dog.

> Strength Training Reminder: Aim for at least 2–3 sessions a week to maintain a strong body. I highly recommend incorporating:
> - Lateral lunges (sideways)
> - Backward lunges
> - Diagonal lunges
> - Hip circles
> - Upper body exercises, like standing movements, bent over T's, and" wall or bench push-ups
> - Scapular squeezes (lots of them) throughout the day.

By including these exercises, you're strengthening your body in all planes of movement—sagittal, frontal, and transverse.

Can I get a double woof? *Woof, woof!*

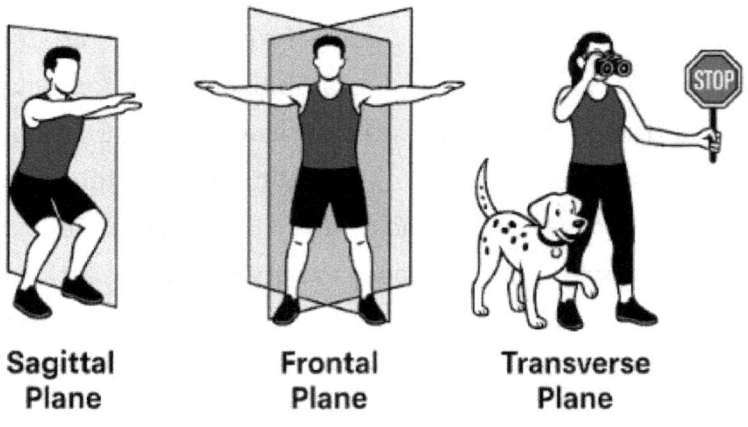

The three planes of movement

Take care of your body, build healthy habits early, and make them a part of your lifestyle. This is where your dog comes in—it's more than just a lifestyle; it's a "dog style," if you will. If you prefer taking your dog to the dog park to burn off energy, that's great! Just be sure to stay active—walk around and do some exercises to take care of your health, too. Think of it as a team effort—you and your dog. Remember, team hound, buds!

If you notice your dog limping, give them time to rest for a while—just like us, dogs can experience muscle strains and ligament sprains too! If they don't improve, take them to the veterinarian.

As for yourself, if you're experiencing aches or something doesn't feel right, seek guidance sooner rather than later. If I had a nickel for every patient who said, "I should've come sooner," my retirement savings would be much larger, for sure! You are your best doctor, at least initially. When you feel "off," experience pain, or just don't feel like your normal self, that's your body's early warning system going off. Listen to it.

I call this athletic awareness—the ability to recognize and understand your body's signals. If you sense something is off, trust that instinct. Ignoring early warning signs can turn minor aches and pains into bigger issues that take much longer to heal. If you don't believe me, just ask your friends—most people wait too long to seek help and regret it.

SAMPLE WORKOUTS

Aim for at least 30 minutes of brisk walking five to seven times a week. Incorporate strength training two to three times a week, and as you age, prioritize stretching and balance exercises most days of the week. Above all, remember the key mantra: Move well and move often. Motion is medicine for your body.

> ### WALKING TIPS TO AVOID INJURIES
>
> - Maintain good posture by keeping your shoulders back and relaxed.
> - Keep your eyes forward to stay aware of your surroundings.
> - Wear comfortable, supportive shoes with good traction, especially in colder climates. Replace them every 300-500 miles or every six months for optimal support.
> - Stay hydrated to maintain energy and prevent fatigue.
> - Be mindful of obstacles, such as tree roots, rocks, uneven sidewalks, slippery surfaces, and dog leashes.

- Wear reflective clothing in low-light conditions for both you and your dog.
- Check the air quality before heading out, as it plays a key role in overall healthy habits.

Understanding both your and your dog's capabilities is key. Everyone is more mature here, and maturity comes with a level of respect. You've built your team, set things in motion, and achieved the level of activity you aimed for—well done, A-team!

The mutual respect between you and your dog is enough to bring happiness to both of you. Just remember to reward yourselves for staying motivated and committed to each other!

TIP #11
MOVEMENT IS MEDICINE.
BUILD YOUR TEAM.

Remember the story of the tortoise and the hare—slow and steady wins the race? This is a metaphor for fitness: Those who are patient, consistent, and put in steady effort will ultimately succeed over those who push too hard.

The careless and feckless hare (e.g., those who push their body into pain) couldn't recover from their blunder (injury). Don't be the hare. I need you to be strong and ready for the battlefield of life. Be the tortoise—steady, smart, and unstoppable!

Be deliberate. Be intentional. Most importantly, be yourself, have fun, and take life slooooooowly. Let your and your dog's bodies gradually adapt to increased movement.

If I haven't drilled it into your cerebral hemisphere yet, *slow and steady wins the race.* This approach will prevent overuse injuries. You'll come out on top, your dog will stay healthy, and your overall well-being will improve safely!

STORY

Imagine a family that makes regular exercise a part of their routine for themselves and their dog. They started with short walks, gradually increasing the distance and incorporating strength exercises. Over time, they noticed significant improvements in their health and fitness, while their dog became more energetic and happier. These shared activities deepened their bond and created lasting memories along the way.

TIP #12
PROGRESS SLOWLY.
RESULTS ARE ACHIEVED.

RECOMMENDATIONS

- Encourage children and adolescents to engage in at least 60 minutes of moderate to vigorous physical activity daily.
- Incorporate muscle-strengthening activities at least three times a week.
- Increase exercise duration and intensity gradually, following the 10 percent rule to prevent injury.

- Watch for signs of pain or discomfort and seek professional help early if needed.
- Provide your dog with a variety of exercises to promote balanced fitness and prevent muscle imbalances.

SUMMARY

Slow and steady wins the race. By gradually increasing physical activity and prioritizing injury prevention, you can maintain a healthy, active lifestyle with your family and your dog. Remember, motion is lotion and medicine for your body. The key to success is consistency over time.

CHAPTER 13

HEALTHIER TOGETHER: EMBRACING ACTIVE LIFESTYLES WITH OUR FURRY FRIENDS

Staying active is essential for maintaining a strong body, improving your quality of life, and avoiding costly treatments for preventable injuries and illnesses as you age. By incorporating movement into your daily routine, you can help foster a healthier, happier community where everyone benefits from shared activity and mutual support.

HUMAN ELEMENT

During our teens and twenties, many of us discover activities we love. Encouraging movement during these years is crucial. If you haven't found a favorite yet, try joining a group, an intramural team, or even finding a walking buddy. For us "dog" people, there are fellow dog lovers in every neighborhood, so don't hesitate to connect with a neighbor. Establishing an *oikos*, a larger family nucleus, helps create a supportive community that cares for one another.

As we enter our thirties, energy levels fluctuate—some feel at their peak while others notice a dip. Regardless, it's essential to keep moving. Newton's first law of inertia reminds us that bodies at rest stay at rest, while those in motion stay in motion. Successful individuals tend to stay active and engaged. Start small, like adding 1,000 extra steps to your daily routine, and let that momentum be your inertial spark to discovering what your body needs to stay healthy and happy.

Maintaining flexibility and strength becomes crucial as we enter our forties and beyond. Simple tasks like reaching for dishes or putting on shoes can become difficult without regular movement. Staying active helps prevent stiffness and weakness, keeping you independent, mobile, and healthy.

DOG CARE

Just like you, your dog needs lifelong guidance and socialization. Your community thrives on mutual support and active engagement with fellow dog lovers. Arrange playdates with vaccinated, friendly dogs in a fenced backyard while you exercise. Do squats, lunges, or jumping jacks as they socialize. It's a win-win —you get a workout, and your dog gets to play!

TIP #13
PRIORITIZE TIME. IT'S A LIFESTYLE.

Regular exercise is essential for both you and your dog. Neglecting your health now may lead to battling illness later. Remember, movement is medicine–don't stagnate.

Too often, we stand around chatting while our dogs play together. Instead, keep the conversation going while adding movement—do a mini-workout, stretch, or take a brisk walk. It's a win-win situation and an efficient use of your time.

Most of us can find the time to be active, especially when we prioritize working out with friends or family. Younger folks, don't forget to visit your parents, grandparents, or even a neighbor and offer to walk their dog. It's a great way to stay active while spending quality time with loved ones. You're welcome, Mom and Dad! Life only gets busier as we age—that's a fact.

Every day you stay active with your furry buddy is a win. These daily victories add up, and your dog's health and happiness depend on you.

Focus on what you can control, such as your attitude, preparation, and effort. Think *carpe diem*—a Latin phrase meaning "seize the day." Take ownership of your well-being. Make time for yourself. Make time for your dog—they rely on you. You are the most important person in your dog's life.

Be the captain of your ship, with your dog as your first mate. Daily wins are key and cumulative! We want wins in life. Every day with your furry buddy is one of those wins. Find your motivation, create inertia, and stack up the wins in your life.

Successful people are often the movers and shakers of the world because they thrive on action; they keep moving and learning and are always on the go. In contrast, others can get stuck, needing a spark of inertia to set them in motion.

Find your spark. Dig deep and create momentum to get yourself moving. Start small—aim for just an extra 1,000 steps a day. That's roughly half a mile and could be the catalyst for building inertia. What will be your spark?

TIP #14
BE THE CAPTAIN. CREATE INERTIA.

SAMPLE WORKOUTS

Try this Dog'ercise routine with your dog:

- Warm-Up: Walk briskly with your dog for 5–10 minutes. This key movement will be repeated throughout the book.
- Goblet Squats: Do 15 reps while your dog runs around outside.
- Lunges: Perform 10 repetitions (reps) per leg while your dog walks beside you.
- Park Bench Push-ups: Complete 10 reps while your dog takes a short rest.
- Cooldown: Walk slowly for 5 minutes, then stretch. Finish by relaxing on a park bench with some positive affirmation while petting your dog.

If you're feeling low on energy, start with the basics: Get sufficient sleep, eat nutritious meals, and move more. The small choices you make throughout the day add up, shaping how you feel and look over time.

To stay limber, include more mobility into your routine—a key area often overlooked and neglected. If you're someone who says, "I've never been flexible," it's likely you haven't made stretching a habit. C'mon! You don't need to be as pliable as Gumby, but maintaining a healthy range of motion is essential for your overall well-being. Trust me—you'll appreciate it later in life!

If you don't maintain flexibility, your body will gradually stiffen, making everyday tasks harder, like reaching up to put dishes away or bending down to put on your shoes. Worse yet, getting up from the floor can be a real challenge if you lack flexibility and strength.

Strengthening your body through a full range of motion is key—you'll only get weaker without it. Keep those joints flexible, stay strong, and maintain full mobility!

EDUCATIONAL INSIGHTS

- Consistency is key: Regular exercise routines benefit you and your dog.
- Add variety: Mix up activities to keep things exciting and work different muscle groups.
- Prioritize safety: Make sure your dog is vaccinated and healthy before playing with other dogs.

STORY

Once upon a time, a woman named Brenda struggled to find time for exercise while juggling work and family life. She decided to include her dog, Alfred, in her routine. They began with short walks, gradually incorporating Dog'ercise sessions in the backyard. Brenda realized that exercising together improved her fitness and deepened her bond with Alfred. Her dedication inspired the neighborhood, and others joined in, creating a vibrant, active community supporting one another's well-being.

Imagine a world where everyone prioritized both their own and their dogs' well-being. Communities would flourish, healthcare costs would decrease, and people would live longer, happier lives. The bond between humans and their dogs would grow stronger, creating a ripple effect of "pawsitivity" and overall wellness. In this world, the joy of shared activity would be a cornerstone of life, fostering connections and cultivating a true sense of belonging.

RECOMMENDATIONS

- Schedule regular exercise sessions with your dog.
- Find a walking buddy or join a group activity.
- Incorporate flexibility and strengthening exercises into your routine.
- Make small, consistent changes to boost daily activity.
- Create a supportive community that values health and wellness.

SUMMARY

Invest in both your and your dog's well-being today for a happier, healthier tomorrow. Regular exercise is crucial for preventing injuries and maintaining overall wellness. By taking small, intentional steps, you can have a positive impact on both your life and the lives of those around you. If you don't make time for physical activity now, you'll be forced to make time for illness later. Motion is lotion—don't be a couch potato! No one will invest in you more than you.

Think of your health like a retirement fund; the choices you make today will compound and have a lasting impact over time. As financial investment grows, so does the return on investing in yourself. That's one stock you can bet on—start now. Invest in yourself and keep growing!

As Jackie Joyner-Kersee once said, "Age is no barrier. It's a limitation you put on your mind." Aging is inevitable, but feeling old is simply a choice.

> *Today is the oldest you've ever been, and the youngest you'll ever be again.*
> *—Eleanor Roosevelt*

CHAPTER 14

AGING ACTIVELY: THE SENIOR YEARS

As we age, injury prevention becomes crucial for maintaining independence and quality of life into our retirement years. Injuries can have more serious consequences as we age, making staying active even more important for us and our dogs. Rest equals rust, and you sure as heck will need a whole lot of lubrication to keep moving!

HUMAN ELEMENT

Your choices will either open doors to new opportunities or close them. Maintaining your independence significantly improves your quality of life, while losing it can have the opposite effect. As the saying goes, "Have a twinkle in your wrinkle,"—embrace aging while becoming the best version of yourself. Congrats on your retirement or semi-retirement! I hope you've taken care of your body so that now it can take great care of you.

A classic dad joke is "I'm fearful of the calendar—its days seem to be numbered." But there's no need to worry about you. You've built a strong, well-oiled, resilient, ready-to-hit-the-slopes iron man body ready to keep up with life's adventures. Now, it's time to grab your dog and explore the world!

Just like a fine wine, you get better with age, but staying active is the key. Retirement doesn't mean rest. Sure, you can relax more—you've earned it—but keep moving and enjoying life!

TIP #15
DRIVE ON. DO NOT RUST.

Have you heard of sarcopenia? It's the natural loss of muscle mass and strength that occurs with aging. This decline increases the risk of falls, fractures, and a lower quality of life. A sedentary lifestyle can accelerate muscle loss, often starting in your forties.[19]

If you don't stay active, you could lose at least 1–5 percent of your muscle mass each decade, significantly impacting mobility and independence. Lose muscle, lose freedom. An injury can take that independence away even faster. Muscles drive movement, and movement helps maintain muscle strength. Staying active is essential to counteract sarcopenia. While staying active together, it's important to customize your exercise routines. Some people thrive on split routines, targeting different muscle groups each day, while others prefer full-body functional movements. Regardless, by moving and being active, the key to long-term success is finding what works best for you and staying consistent.

---

[19] Volpi, Edoardo, R. Nazemi, and S. Fujita. "Muscle Tissue Changes with Aging." *Current Opinion in Clinical Nutrition* and Metabolic Care." 7, no. 4 (2004): 405-410.

THE IMPORTANCE OF STRETCHING

One of my favorite activities? Stretching. Yes, you heard me right! Stretching has been a part of my life since my younger years in tae kwon do, inspired by Jean-Claude Van Damme movies, or was it my introduction to fitness through Denise Austin workouts? Either way, I learned that stretching is fantastic for your body. Looking back, I appreciate my high school coach's emphasis on stretching—thank you, coach! Their guidance has reinforced this habit and, over the years, has helped me prevent injuries and stay active.

Do you know who else stretches daily? Elite athletes, including one of the greatest quarterbacks of all time, Tom Brady, also known as the greatest of all time (GOAT). I've read he relies on muscle pliability training, stretching, and foam rolling to keep his muscles primed. "What does it mean to be primed?" you ask. It's the ability to continuously perform at an elite level, allowing muscles to absorb and disperse stress effectively—a key factor in avoiding injuries. This approach aligns perfectly with my belief that maintaining a full range of motion in your joints helps prevent future problems. No, the GOAT hasn't officially endorsed this, but I'm sure he'd happily autograph a Dog'ercise book for a fan. That's good enough for me!

Stretching ensures your joints move through their full range of motion, improving overall performance. Being stiff or restricted can hinder movement and increase your risk of injury. Stiffness reduces your muscles' ability to absorb forces, making you more vulnerable to muscle strains or even tears. It's simple: If your muscles move better, you feel better. If you've ever had a muscle knot, you know exactly what I'm talking about, which is all of us at some point!

Pliability is the crucial missing leg that will complete and complement our workouts.
—Tom Brady a.k.a. the GOAT

Make sure you are pliable, malleable, limber, supple, and flexible—all terms that relate to having the right tissue length and mobility for your activities. The more you work on your movement, the more resilient you become.

Think of it like sweetgrass. Huh? If you've ever woven baskets made of sweetgrass (I'm sure *many* of you have, right?), you know what I'm talking about. This grass's long, durable blades bend easily, are highly flexible, and can withstand whatever Mother Nature throws their way.

That's what pliability is all about—bending without breaking, folks. Plus, sweetgrass smells like vanilla and warm hay, which has nothing to do with stretching, but hey, it's an added bonus. Bottom line: Stretching is powerful, I doggone guarantee it!

Avoid being too rigid in movement and in life. Like most things, stretching is subject to debate, but it ultimately boils down to proper technique, form, and timing. The best time to stretch? After warming up. Even if you do some light stretching in the morning, you'll see greater benefits when your muscles are warm and loose. That being said, something as simple as walking around the house before stretching can help loosen you up and make your stretches more effective. Some folks are naturally flexible—I'm in that category. If you're hypermobile (meaning your joints move beyond their normal range of motion), it's best to focus on building strength and stability rather than stretching. However, I strongly recommend the stretching exercises I've covered in this book for most people. The key is understanding that exercise isn't one-size-fits-all. Your individual goals, physical condition, and natural flexibility should guide your approach.

Here's a summary of the key points:

- Importance of Proper Form and Timing: Stretching should be done correctly to maximize benefits and prevent injury.
- Stretching After Warming Up: It's best to warm up before deep stretching to improve blood flow, make muscles more pliable, and reduce the risk of injury.
- Morning Stretching versus Post-Warm-Up Stretching: Morning stretches help with wakefulness and general flexibility, but warm-up stretching is better for increasing range of motion.
- Walking as a Warm-up: I recommend a simple warm-up, like walking around the house, before stretching. Low-intensity activities like walking gradually raise your heart rate and prepare your body for more intense exercise.
- Consideration for Hypermobile Individuals: Those with excessive joint mobility (hypermobility) should focus more on strengthening rather than additional stretching.
- Stretching for Most People: Stretching enhances flexibility, joint health, and posture while also reducing muscle stiffness. Moreover, maintaining flexibility decreases fragility and can save you thousands in medical expenses from avoidable injuries!

If you've ever experienced back pain, like many people do at some point, stretching can help keep your spine moving properly. Motion is lotion for the small spinal joints and the long muscles running from the lower back to the head. Yes, these muscles are that long, and there are many of them. They're called erector spinae muscles, also known as postural muscles, and they keep you upright. Regular stretching improves the mobility of this system.

Beneath these muscles lies the myofascial system, an interwoven, tacky layer of connective tissue. Think of it like the thin inner film of a hard-boiled egg—an essential layer that links and integrates everything throughout your entire body. That is excellent!

Imagine a highway crash—one muscle knot or area of tightness can back everything up, creating a bottleneck of poor movement and discomfort. I'd rather have clear roads with free-flowing traffic. Do you think stretching is important now? I'd say so!

In physical therapy, restoring joint motion is always a top priority, whether recovering from an injury or post-surgery. Before addressing the strength or other system components, we must first ensure proper movement. "Why?" you ask. Because strengthening a dysfunctional muscle makes no sense. Remember, the quality of movement is key. This is where stretching plays a crucial role—helping to restore the full range of motion in the tissues and joints before adding strength. The goal is to allow your muscles to function at their ideal length without overloading other muscles or structures. With time, this could lead to an injury.

For me, quality motion is the only standard operating procedure (SOP) I follow, and a good PT can also help. Once you move well, move often. That's been the message throughout this book.

Well, what about our dogs? Of course, stretching applies to them too—why wouldn't it? If you watch your dog wake up from a siesta, notice how they instinctively stretch, often striking a yoga-like pose. Not as frequently as our cat friends, but this prepares their bodies for action. It's built into all of us. My vizslas are masters of the downward dog, doing it all the time. And no, I didn't train them to do it—though occasionally I take the credit!

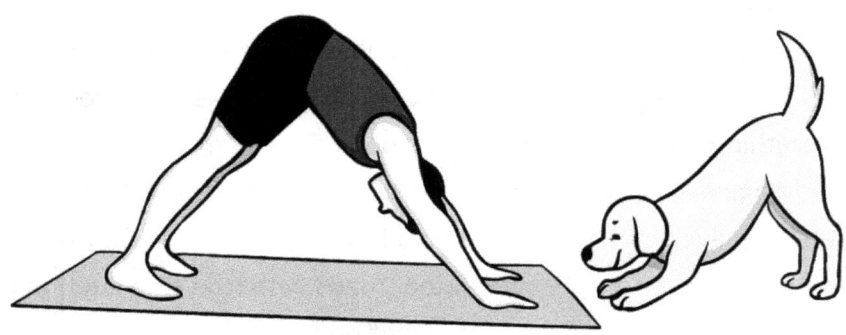

"Doga" in action—do the downward dog!

Naturally, downward dog is a great stretch—it's incredibly beneficial, just like all the other stretches we've discussed. Some refer to this as the "greeting stretch," where the front legs extend forward while the hips stay high. Other dogs *sploot*, which is darn adorable. Splooting is slang for our furry friends lying flat on their belly and rear legs stretched out. Corgis and shih tzus are always prone to this—it's darling! This is one example of people and dogs will naturally do things that just feel good.

If you don't know what I'm talking about, search for images of dog splooting and get ready to laugh. Just like many different stretching positions, there are various including the full sploot, superman sploot, cross-legged sploot, half or quarter sploot, the infamous side sploot, and the rolling sploot. Dogs love to stretch out, and splooting helps improve hip flexibility, provides a comfortable position for relaxation, and aids in cooling the body quickly. My shih tzu would naturally find a poodle of water to sploot in. Most of the time, it was a mud puddle. *Woof!*

If your dog doesn't naturally stretch themselves, take a few minutes to gently help them slowly move their limbs. Be patient—never force or rush the stretch. While you're at it, throw in a few belly rubs and ear scratches; it's quality time together, and you'll be helping them stay limber and relaxed.

SAMPLE STRETCHING ROUTINE

Once warmed up, aim for 60 seconds of total stretch time for each tissue group to achieve an effective stretch. If mobility is limited, increase the stretch time and repeat several times a day until you achieve your desired range of motion. Find the routine that works for you and supports your movement needs. Avoid pushing too hard or bouncing into discomfort. Remember—a dose of stretching a day helps keep the PT away!

BALANCE

Simple balance exercises like standing on one leg can be easily incorporated into daily activities. Good balance keeps us steady on our feet.

THE COST OF FALLS

Falls can be costly and potentially life-altering, particularly for older adults. Below are some sample figures illustrating the potential financial impact of falls among older adults. It's important to note that these costs vary widely depending on location, healthcare systems, personal circumstances, and other factors. At the time of printing, these figures are approximate and expressed in US dollars; actual costs may differ based on individual situations:

Physical injuries:
- Hip fracture surgery: $30,000–$40,000+
- Rehabilitation costs: $10,000–$20,000+

Hospitalization and medical expenses:
- Emergency room visit: $1,000–$3,000+
- Hospital stays for a fracture: $20,000–$40,000+

Decreased quality of life:
- Physical therapy sessions: $100–$200 per session
- Assistive devices, e.g., walker, cane: $50–$500+

Functional decline:
- Home modifications, e.g., grab bars, ramps: $1,000–$5,000+
- In-home care services: $20–$30+ per hour

Increased healthcare utilization:
- Doctor visits and follow-up appointments: $100–$300+ per visit
- Medication costs: Varies depending on prescriptions

Psychological impact:
- Counseling or therapy sessions: $50–$150+ per session
- Medications for anxiety or depression: Varies widely

Caregiver burden:
- Additional home care services: $20–$30+ per hour
- Potential loss of income for caregivers: Varies based on employment

Institutionalization:
- Assisted living facility: $3,000–$6,000+ per month
- Nursing home care: $7,000–$10,000+ per month

TOTAL COST: $75,000–$125,000+

Need I say more? Falls are expensive! This should be enough motivation to prioritize balance training—otherwise, you might be saying goodbye to your hard-earned retirement savings. As we age, balance naturally declines, making it paramount to incorporate balance exercises into our regular routines.

According to the CDC, one in four people over the age of 65 experiences a fall each year.[20] That's not good! I highly recommend checking out the CDC's resources on fall prevention for olderadults. They provide valuable information to help keep your aging athletes—yes, I said athletes—safe and active. Aren't we all athletes? I like to think so—so should you.

---

[20] Volpi, Nazemi, and Fujita, "Muscle Tissue," 405-10.

PREVENTING FALLS:
A PHYSICAL THERAPIST'S PERSPECTIVE

How can we reduce the risk of falls? From a physical therapy standpoint, balance exercises play a key role in improving reaction time—the speed at which your nervous system and muscles communicate to correct a misstep.

When reaction time slows down, the risk of falling increases significantly, resulting in a higher likelihood of injuries. The solution? Strong bones, a well-conditioned muscular system, and quicker reaction time. Prioritizing these will help prevent falls and protect against fractures.

RULES FOR BETTER BALANCE

- Check Your Medications: Some medications can cause lightheadedness, dizziness, or fogginess.
- Make Sure Your Vision is GTG—Good to go! If you can't see a darn thing, that's a problem—get your eyes checked!
- Improve Nighttime Safety: Most falls happen at night while walking from the bedroom to the bathroom. Use night lights, people! I don't want you tripping over your dog or their bed during the night.
- Eliminate Household Hazards: Reduce tripping risks by removing loose rugs or fixing damaged floors (yes, I have seen holes in floors).
- Encourage your dog to avoid lying in high-traffic areas.

The biggest key to better balance? Drum roll, please—stay active, strengthen your muscles, and practice balance exercises! I can read your mind—I'm sensing you're thinking, "But Brandon, what balance exercises should I do?" Try these:

SAMPLE BALANCE ROUTINE

- Keep it Simple: Set aside 1-2 minutes most days of the week to practice single-leg balance. Easy peasy, lemon squeezy!
- Another option? Hold a 10-second balance here, 30 seconds there—consistency is key.

Too easy!

SOME BALANCING TIPS:

- Waiting for food to heat up in the microwave? Practice balancing!
- Brushing your teeth? Practice more balancing!
- Feeling advanced? Try balancing in an elevator or on an escalator.

Be creative. Don't be bored with this—boredom only happens when your mind isn't engaged.

Test Your Balance: What's your baseline?

First things first—stand up. Seriously. Do it now! Are you standing yet? Waiting. Finally, thank you! Now let's safely test your balance:

- Stand near a countertop for support if needed.
- Start with your eyes open—always begin here before advancing.
- Can you balance on your left leg? How about your right leg?

Time yourself and track your progress year after year to measure your improvement over time.

Now, how about trying it with your eyes closed? Whoa, pappy—master the eyes-open version first! This will amplify the difficulty by removing a key sensory input. Mama Mia!

Try this single-leg balance test with your eyes open. Aim to be consistent with both legs.

SCORE:

- 5 seconds: Average—Not bad! A solid start.
- 10 seconds: Bronze medal—You're making progress!
- 30 seconds: Silver medal—Nice job!
- 1 minute or greater—Bling, bling, you're holding the gold medal, champion!

Where did you land? (see what I did there?)

These guidelines are general, not strict scientific benchmarks. If you're competitive (and I know many of you are!), I say go for the gold!

If one leg is harder to balance on than the other, spend extra time strengthening that side to even things out. We want a stable footing, not a peg leg!

Better balance equals better vitality, I say. If you can improve your balance, I bet you'll have better vitality. It just makes sense.

If this activity challenges you, don't stress! Balance, like any skill, can be improved with practice.

PROGRESSION STEPS TO BUILD BALANCE:

- If you can't balance on one leg quite yet, start with both feet on the ground. Bring them close together to narrow your base of support—this increases the challenge.
- Next, progress to a wider staggered stance (position one foot slightly offset from the other foot). As this improves, transition to a narrower staggered stance.
- Advance to a tandem stance (heel-to-toe, like walking a tight rope).
- Once you're stable in the tandem stance, progress to single-leg balancing.

DOG CARE

Just like humans, dogs thrive with regular exercise. It helps them maintain a healthy weight, build muscles, and improve overall well-being. Incorporating your dog into your balance workout is a fun and effective way to keep both of you active and engaged. I've even slow-danced with my dog, gently holding their front paws.

Keeping your dog engaged in activities like fetching, running, and agility training helps keep them mentally and physically fit. For older dogs or those with joint issues, low-impact exercises like swimming are excellent alternatives. Regular exercise prevents behavioral problems and promotes a longer, healthier life.

INJURY PREVENTION FOR DOGS

Follow these key injury prevention tips to keep your dog safe and healthy:

- Schedule regular vet checkups to monitor their well-being.
- Warm up before strenuous activities.
- Use appropriate gear such as well-fitted harnesses and sturdy leashes.
- Keep their nails trimmed to prevent slipping.
- Provide a balanced diet to support overall health.

SAMPLE WORKOUTS

Strength Training: Full-body, functional compound movements engage multiple muscles and joints across different planes to create desired movements. (See Chapter 12) I prefer doing these because they mimic real-life activities.

Incorporate this routine 2–3 times a week to improve your balance and strength:

Time commitment: 15–30 minutes

- Exercises: 4–6 functional exercises that engage multiple muscle groups.
- Sets: 1–3 sets, depending on your time availability.
- Repetitions (reps): 6–15 on average.

Your effort or intensity should match your weight selection and rep range, based on your goal. On some days, I focus on strength by lifting heavier weights, aiming for around 6 reps to activate fast-twitch muscle fibers. Other days, I prioritize endurance, performing 15 or more reps with lighter weights to build stamina.

There's no one-size-fits-all approach—find out what works for you!

Experts recommend a periodization program for high school, college, or elite athletes. This structured training plan helps athletes optimize performance by adjusting training cycles accordingly. However, for most of us just aiming for healthy aging, the key theme is to keep moving.

Use this simplified guide to adjust your repetition range. Feel free to mix it up to engage all muscle fibers for strength, muscle growth, or endurance, setting yourself up for success!

- Muscle Strength: 4-6 reps
- Muscle Growth: 8-14 reps
- Muscle Endurance: 15+ reps

Incorporate your dog into your workout routine with these fun exercises:

- Lunges with Controlled Upper Body Rotation: Hold your dog (if they are small enough) or use a weight while performing lunges.
- Walking Lunges: Walk with lunges, allowing your dog to walk alongside or carry a small dog for added resistance.
- Side Lunges with Arms Out: Extend your arms for balance while lunging to the side.

- Push-ups with Slow, Controlled Movements: Perform push-ups with your dog lying nearby for moral support.
- Jumping Jacks and Burpees: Include your dog in the fun by encouraging them to jump around or follow your movements.
- Squats: Hold your dog or a weight while performing squats.

EDUCATIONAL INSIGHTS

- Regular Vet Checkups: Schedule routine veterinary visits.
- Proper Nutrition: Provide a well-balanced diet tailored to your dog's age, size, and activity level.
- Joint Health: Consider supplements like glucosamine and chondroitin to support joint health.
- Warm-up and Cooldown: Just like us, dogs need to warm up before exercise and cool down afterward.
- Hydration: Keep your dog hydrated, especially before, during, and after exercise.

STORY

Cooper, a spirited golden retriever, and his owner, Lilly, have been exercising together for years—hiking, running, and swimming side-by-side. One day, Cooper injured his paw, and Lilly realized the importance of proper warm-ups and cooldowns in their routine. Determined to keep Cooper healthy, she adjusted their workouts to include joint-friendly exercises and slower warm-ups, ensuring Cooper's health was always a priority. Today, Cooper is healthier and happier than ever, proving that a little attention and smart adjustments can go a long way in preventing injuries.

Imagine Jane, a 55-year-old woman who loves hiking with her dog, Bella. One day, Jane slips and falls, breaking her hip. The medical bills pile up, and Jane's independence is suddenly compromised. This accident may have been prevented with regular strength training to build stronger bones and balance exercises to improve reaction time. Now, Jane is determined to regain her strength and never let her independence slip away again. This story highlights the emotional and financial costs of neglecting injury prevention.

RECOMMENDATIONS

- Incorporate Strength Training: Perform strength exercises at least twice a week.
- Practice Balancing Exercises: Include daily balance training to prevent falls.
- Stretch Regularly: Stretch after warming up to improve flexibility and prevent injuries.
- Exercise with Your Dog: Include your dog in your exercise routine for added fun.
- Monitor Your Dog's Health: Regular veterinary checkups, proper nutrition, and joint health support are essential.

SUMMARY

Don't count the days, make the days count.
—Muhammad Ali

Aging well means maintaining physical and mental strength. By prioritizing regular exercise, proper nutrition, and injury prevention, we can ensure a healthier, happier future for both ourselves and our furry friends. Keep moving, stay strong, and enjoy the journey. Do what works for your body, your schedule, and what keeps you motivated, but make sure to include strengthening exercises 2-3 times a week. Make each strengthening day a priority. Prevent the sarcopenia. Explore creative ways to stay active with Dog'ercise.

> **SUMMARY OF SAMPLE EXERCISES**
> **HUMANS**
>
> Activity: Aim for at least 30 minutes of brisk walking most days of the week, and perform strengthening exercises several days a week. Movement is medicine for your body.
>
> Strength: Perform 4–6 functional exercises to target various muscle groups. Do 1–3 sets, depending on the time you have. Include a variety of repetitions to train your muscles, ranging from 3–20 reps. Build your armor.
>
> Balance: This can be as simple as setting aside 1–2 minutes every day. Another option is to add in 10 seconds here, 30 seconds there—in other words, sporadically throughout the day. Easy peasy, lemon squeezy!
>
> Stretching: After warming up, stretch each muscle group for 60 seconds. If your movement is limited, increase your total time several times daily to reach your desired motion.

You'll find the routine that your body responds to and needs. Be pliable, and a daily dose helps keep the PT away.

DOGS

Know your breed. At a minimum, aim for 60 minutes of daily activity, whether playtime, walking, or a combination. Move is a four-legged word. Break up this total time for your older dogs into smaller increments throughout the day.

CHAPTER 15

THE TEMPLE: MOVE WELL, LIVE WELL

Our bodies are our temples, and staying injury-free allows us to move freely and live fully. Prevention is key—not just for physical health, but also for financial well-being. Regular exercise benefits both the body and mind, improving quality of life. This chapter explores the importance of movement for both humans and dogs, providing practical tips and examples to protect our temples.

At first glance, the most obvious difference between humans and dogs is how we move—humans walk upright (meaning we're bipedal, the fancy medical term for walking on two feet), while our furry friends move on all fours, making them quadrupedal. Other than that, we're not so different—we both have muscles, bones, a nervous system, a heart, skin, and internal organs, among some other things. We're built to move—no matter how many legs we have!

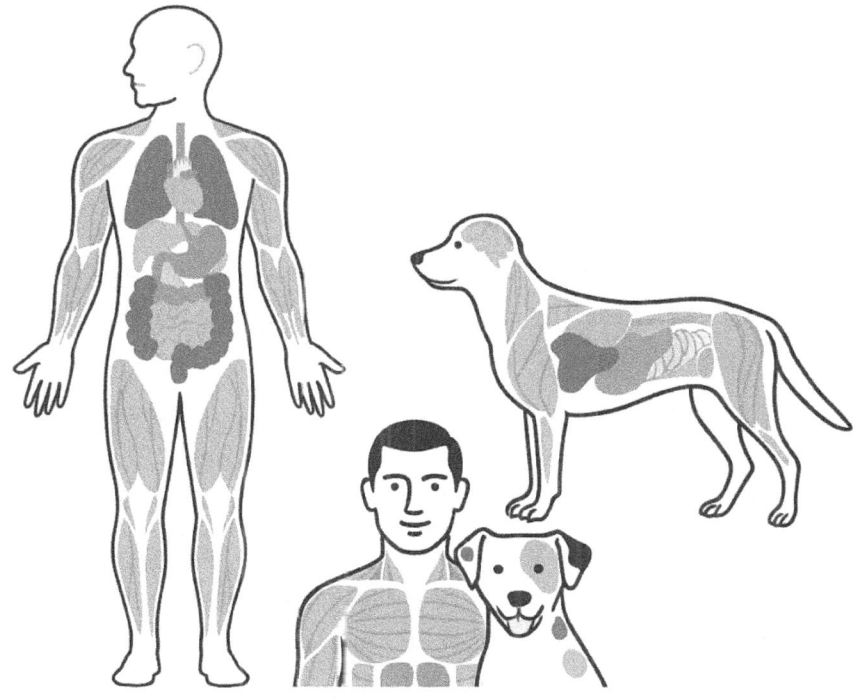

We're not so different; we're all built to move!

TIP #16
MOVE. MAINTAIN INERTIA.

HUMAN ELEMENT

Movement is essential for maintaining muscle strength and health. Regular physical activity improves blood flow and oxygen delivery, thereby supporting cognitive function and mental clarity. Additionally, movement lubricates joints and cartilage, reducing the risk of arthritis and other joint-related issues. The benefits don't stop there—exercise also boosts emotional well-being, reducing anxiety, depression, and stress while enhancing mood and overall mental health.

Some other great things that exercise can do for us:

- Stronger Bones and Reduced Health Risks: Regular exercise helps strengthen bones, thereby reducing the risk of osteoporosis and fractures. Maintaining a healthy weight also reduces the risk of heart disease, strokes, type 2 diabetes, cancer, and high blood pressure.
- Better Sleep and Stress Management: Staying active improves sleep quality and increases resilience, making it easier to handle stress and enhancing our overall wellness.
- Over 600 Muscles at Work: The human body has hundreds of muscles, enabling us to perform a wide range of activities and movements.
- Hearts that Work Hard: Our hearts beat over 100,000 times a day, and regular exercise makes them more efficient at pumping blood.

TIP #17
KNOW THY BODY.
MARVEL AND APPRECIATE.

DOG CARE

Just like humans, dogs benefit immensely from regular movement. Exercise keeps their muscles and joints healthy, reducing the risk of conditions like arthritis. Physical activity strengthens the heart, keeping it strong and working efficiently. Additionally, regular movement helps reduce anxiety and boosts their mood.

- Maintain a Healthy Weight: Regular exercise helps prevent obesity-related health issues.
- Boosts Immunity: An active lifestyle strengthens the immune system, leading to fewer illnesses and a longer, healthier life.
- Supports Strong Bones and Injury Prevention: Movement helps maintain bone strength, reduces the risk of injuries, and ensures our furry friends stay active.

FUN DOG FACTS

- Dogs have eighteen muscles in their ears, allowing them to fine-tune their hearing to detect sounds more effectively in their surroundings.
- A Beating Heart: A dog's heart can beat up to 150,000 times a day, with larger breeds typically having lower heart rates.
- Super Sniffers: A dog's sense of smell is up to 100,000 times more powerful than a human's.

Where does a dog shop when it loses its tail? A retail store!

As you can see, movement benefits our bodies, humans, and dogs alike! The keyword in all exercises is *movement*. Let's move better together! Forward propulsion. Jet setting. Wheels spinning. Pedal to the metal. Onward and upward. Taking it to the next level. Driving on. Pushing on. Elevate. Make headway. One step at a time. You get it. All phrases to help us maintain movement—inertia. Let's take a look at what movement does for us. Rev up your engines—here comes a poem!

> "Dance, Dog, Dance!"
> At long last, move well, my little troops.
> I want you to grow into your big boots.
> Make sure to dance and move.
> Have fun while you shake and groove.
> Remember to make a strong caboose.

Why do we need movement?

- It Strengthens the Muscles and Heart: Movement keeps our muscles strong, including our hearts, so we can explore the world. Yes, your heart is a muscle—*thump-thump, lub-dub*.
- Sharpens the Mind: Movement improves blood flow, delivering oxygen and feel-good hormones to our brain and body. Stay mentally sharp!
- Lubricates Joints and Cartilage: Motion is lotion.
- Keeps Instincts Strong: Movement fuels our natural instincts, including those birds and bees moments.
- Boosts Mood and Energy: Movement brings peace of mind, lifts your mood, and increases energy. Namaste.
- Improves Mental Health: Regular physical activity reduces anxiety and depression, and helps keep your sense of humor.
- Strengthens Bones: Remember Wolff's Law.
- Supports Healthy Weight and Longevity: Staying active helps maintain a healthy weight and promotes a longer lifespan.

- Lowers Health Risks: Regular physical activity reduces the risk of numerous health issues, including heart disease, stroke, type 2 diabetes, cancer, arthritis, and high blood pressure. Stay vigorous!
- Improves Sleep: Movement during the day helps you sleep better at night—lights out, nighty night!
- Builds Resilience: Movement helps your body better handle stress. Stay robust!
- Boosts Immunity: Regular activity strengthens your immune system, leading to fewer sick days—and that's an economic boost!
- It Keeps You Healthy: At the end of the day, movement equals health. That's the take-home message!

SAMPLE WORKOUTS

Engage in activities that both you and your dog can enjoy together. Examples include:

- Walking or Running: A simple and effective way to get moving.
- Fetch Games: Incorporate running and agility exercises.
- Agility Training: Set up an obstacle course to challenge your coordination.
- Swimming: A fantastic full-body workout that's easy on the joints.

EDUCATIONAL INSIGHTS

- Know Thy Dog: Understand your dog's physical limits and health needs to ensure safe exercise.
- Schedule Regular Veterinary Checkups: Ensure your dog is healthy and fit for exercise.
- Provide Proper Nutrition: A balanced diet supports their energy levels and overall well-being.

STORY

Bella, a lively Labrador retriever, once loved to play but began slowing down due to weight gain and joint pain. Her owner, Mark, decided to act. They started with short, daily walks, gradually adding fetch games and agility exercises. As Bella's activity level increased, her weight dropped, joint pain decreased, and her energy returned. Mark also noticed positive changes in his own health, including improved stamina and a better mood. Their shared fitness journey transformed their physical well-being and strengthened their bond, demonstrating the power of regular exercise for humans and dogs.

Imagine a world where every human and dog stayed active. Obesity rates would plummet, healthcare costs would drop, and overall happiness and well-being would soar. Communities would be more active and connected, creating a healthier, vibrant society.

RECOMMENDATIONS

- Set a Routine: Schedule regular exercise sessions to keep you and your dog active.
- Track Progress: Monitor improvements and adjust routines as needed.
- Stay Informed: Keep up to date with the latest exercise and health guidelines from trusted sources like the CDC and ACSM.
- Keep it Fun: Incorporate a variety of activities to keep exercise engaging and fun.

SUMMARY

Movement is a medicine for creating change in a person's physical, emotional, and mental states.
—Carol Welch

By prioritizing regular exercise for both ourselves and our dogs, we can build stronger, healthier bodies while deepening our bond with our furry companions. Embrace the journey to better health and well-being, one step at a time!

CHAPTER 16:

CREATING A ROADMAP: EXERCISE ROUTINES FOR YOU AND YOUR DOG

Injury prevention is not just about avoiding pain and discomfort; it's also a savvy way to save money. Medical bills, lost workdays, and decreased productivity can add up quickly when injuries occur. We can significantly reduce the risk of injuries by adopting regular exercise routines for ourselves and our dogs. This is why establishing a battle rhythm, otherwise known as a roadmap, is important. This means establishing a set of guidelines and a day-to-day routine that you can consistently follow. This proactive approach enhances our quality of life and ensures our furry friends stay healthy and happy.

HUMAN ELEMENT

Fitting exercise into a busy schedule can be challenging. Start small with just 5–10 minutes of exercise daily, gradually increasing to 30 minutes five to six days a week. Be consistent. The key to success is finding a routine that fits your lifestyle and commitments. Whether it's a morning jog, lunchtime walk, or evening yoga session, incorporating exercise as a regular part of your day can have profound benefits.

DOG CARE

It's important to tailor your dog's exercise routine based on their individual needs to avoid injury. Every dog has unique exercise needs, based on their breed, age, and health. Working breeds and young dogs typically need more frequent and vigorous exercise, while older dogs or those with health issues may require gentler, low-impact activities.

Incorporating play into your dog's exercise routine makes staying active fun and engaging for both of you. Fetch, agility training, or a simple walk in the park are great ways to keep your dog active. These sessions strengthen your bond, turning exercise into a shared, enjoyable experience that deepens your connection with your buddy.

SAMPLE WORKOUTS

Dog'ercise blends human workouts with engaging activities for your dog. A typical session might include:

- A warm-up walk to get moving.
- Mix in jogging or running intervals to enhance endurance.
- Incorporate play breaks—try fetch or practicing commands.
- Make it interactive—play a game like tag or hide-and-seek (indoors or outdoors).

- Use healthy dog snacks as motivation and rewards.

This routine keeps you fit while ensuring your dog gets the physical exercise and mental stimulation they need.

EDUCATIONAL INSIGHTS

Dogs thrive on consistency—structured daily routines help them feel secure, reduce anxiety, and reinforce good behavior. Set regular times for meals, walks and exercise, play, and rest. Remember, a well-exercised dog is usually a well-behaved dog.

STORY

Once, a family had a hyperactive border collie named Ace. His boundless energy led to chewed furniture, a dug-up garden, and constant mischief. Determined to find a solution, the family established a structured exercise routine that included daily runs and agility training. Within weeks, Ace's behavior transformed; he became happier, calmer, and more obedient. The family soon realized that Ace's mischievous behavior was a result of pent-up energy and boredom. This experience taught them a valuable lesson: Regular exercise is essential for their dog's mental and physical well-being.

Imagine coming home after a long, exhausting day at work, feeling stressed and drained. Your dog, however, is full of energy, eager for attention. Instead of collapsing on the couch, you grab the leash and head outside. As you stroll through the neighborhood, fresh air and movement help clear your mind, ease tension, and relax your body. Your dog, happy and content, trots beside you. This simple routine not only lifts your mood but also strengthens your bond with your pet. A small effort with big rewards—for both of you.

RECOMMENDATIONS

- Set Realistic Goals: Start with small, achievable exercise goals for you and your dog. Gradually increase the duration and intensity over time.
- Create a Weekly Plan: Dedicate a specific day to map out your exercise schedule, ensuring both you and your dog stay active.
- Stay Flexible: Life is unpredictable, so allow flexibility in your routine while prioritizing movement.
- Commit to Consistency: Whether you prefer a structured schedule or a more flexible approach, sticking with it is key to long-term success.
- Track Progress: Keep a log of your activities, improvements, and milestones. Celebrate progress and adjust goals as needed.
- Build a Routine That Works: A routine is simply a series of consistent actions that help you achieve your goals. This means creating a schedule that fits your lifestyle and committing to it for exercise. Consider your job, responsibilities, and your dog's needs when creating your exercise schedule. Start small and realistic, gradually increasing frequency and duration.

The goal is to make movement a regular, enjoyable part of your life.

TIP #18
CREATE A ROADMAP.
ESTABLISH A ROUTINE.

Design a daily or weekly schedule that includes exercise, play, and rest. This structure helps you manage time effectively, reduce stress, and ensure both you and your dog stay healthy and happy. Remember, flexibility and consistency are the keys to a successful routine.

SUMMARY

Creating a consistent exercise routine for you and your dog helps prevent injuries and enhances overall well-being. A healthy routine is the foundation of a happier, more active life. Be battle-ready and establish your roadmap.

Get free downloadable copies of the Weekly Battle Rhythm Schedule at www.movebettertogether.com.

WEEKLY BATTLE RHYTHM SCHEDULE

Monday	Dog Walk/Playtime/Fitness:	Tuesday
	Family:	
Wednesday	Dog Walk/Playtime/Fitness:	Thursday
	Family:	
Friday	Dog Walk/Playtime/Fitness:	Saturday
	Family:	
Sunday: Plan the week.	Dog Walk/Playtime/Fitness:	Notes:
	Family:	Goals:

Get free downloadable copies at www.movebettertogether.com.

CHAPTER 17

HEEL: PROACTIVE PARTNERSHIP

I use *heel* as a proverbial pause—a crucial moment of control we need with our canine companions. This command can sometimes save lives by preventing dogs from getting into mischief or entering dangerous situations.

HUMAN ELEMENT

- *Heel* is a Reset: A verbal cue that demands immediate attention and focus.
- A Tool for Obedience and Training: Used in performances, competitions, and everyday safety.
- Encourages Self-Awareness: Helps your dog stay aware of their surroundings and maintain proximity to you.

Just as looking both ways before crossing the street, pausing to assess before proceeding is key for both humans and dogs.

Regular exercise is a cornerstone of injury prevention, but maintaining consistency is crucial. If you've fallen off track, it's time to heel—pause, reset, and prioritize your health. So how much exercise do we need? Let's review: Most adults should aim for 150 minutes of moderate-intensity aerobic activity, e.g., brisk walking each week OR 75 minutes of vigorous activity like running each week to support cardiovascular health. Additionally, *ACSM's Guidelines for Exercise Testing and Prescription* recommends strength training at least twice a week. Similarly, the CDC reports that regular physical activity offers a wide range of health benefits, including a reduced risk of chronic diseases, such as heart disease, type 2 diabetes, and certain types of cancer. It also supports weight management and improves mental health."[21]

Preventing injuries isn't just about taking precautions while you're exercising—it also requires proper warm-up and cooldown routines. Heel and make sure you don't skip these essential steps. A thorough warm-up increases blood flow to muscles, reducing stiffness and preparing your body for movement. Cooling down also gradually lowers heart rate and stretches muscles, helping to prevent soreness, stiffness, and injuries. A study in the *Journal of Clinical Psychiatry* found that exercise can be as effective as medication in reducing symptoms of depression and anxiety.[22]

> ### *HEEL* NOW!
>
> If you don't *heel*, you increase your risk of injury. Injuries can be costly—not just in extreme cases like getting hit by a car, but also from everyday accidents like rolling

---

[21] American College of Sports Medicine. *ACSM's Guidelines for Exercise Testing and Prescription*, 11th ed. Wolters Kluwer, 2023; Centers for Disease Control and Prevention. 2025. "Benefits of Physical Activity." Accessed March 23, 2025. https://www.cdc.gov/physical-activity-basics/benefits/index.html

[22] Blumenthal, James A., et al. "Exercise and Pharmacotherapy in the Treatment of Major Depressive Disorder." *Journal of Clinical Psychiatry* 68, no. 5 (2007): 667-76.

> your ankle or tripping and hitting your head on a curb. However, the hidden costs of an injury can be even more burdensome. Beyond medical expenses, injuries can limit your independence, forcing you to rely on others for help. This can lead to feelings of guilt, knowing that your need for assistance might create financial strain, lost work time, or additional responsibilities like household chores or yard work. If you're a caregiver to your kids, parents, or anyone else, an injury can complicate your ability to manage those duties. In these situations, thinking creatively and seeking alternative support systems becomes essential.

Spending time in and around water is joyful and a great exercise for you and your friend. Swimming reduces stress on your joints by providing buoyancy, minimizing impact on your joints, and engaging most of your muscles through resistance and a full range of motion! Before you dive in, *heel*—pause and ensure safety for you and your water dog. Many dogs enjoy splashing around and jumping into the water, but safety comes first. And don't forget grandma's advice: *"Sonny, you need to wait thirty minutes after you eat before you swim."*

While it's true that resting after eating is important (blood flow increases to your digestive system), the amount of rest needed depends on your activity level. Swimming like an Olympian is a high-intensity exercise that requires more rest (digestion time) before jumping in. With lighter activities like floating, you can get in the water sooner. Just like you, your dog also needs a brief rest period after eating before exercising.

TIP #19
BE WISE. PROCEED SAFELY.

DOG CARE

Heat exhaustion is a significant risk to active dogs, particularly in hot weather. Always bring water to keep your dog safe—you can't always rely on public water sources.

Signs of Dehydration in Dogs:

- Excessive panting: Tongue hanging out excessively
- Confusion: Not following commands
- Weakness: Slowing down or struggling to move
- Severe Cases: Collapse or loss of coordination

If you're more active, bring more water. Bring extra water and a collapsible drinking bowl on hot days, and use them frequently. If you're thirsty, your dog will be thirsty too.

Take frequent breaks. A study in *Frontiers in Veterinary Science* found that certain dogs are more prone to heat-related illnesses:

- Brachycephalic (short-nosed) breeds like shih tzus, bulldogs, and boxers struggle to expel heat efficiently due to ineffective panting (my first dog, a shih tzu, was always thirsty).
- Dogs weighing over 110 pounds retain more heat and require extra hydration.[23]

---

[23] Hall, E. J., A. J Carter, and D. G., O'Neill. "Incidence and Risk Factors for Heat-Related Illness (Heatstroke) in UK Dogs under Primary Veterinary Care in 2016." *Frontiers in Veterinary Science* 7 (2020): 491.

Protecting your dog's paws from hot pavement, rough terrain, and icy conditions is important. Consider using dog booties or gradually toughening their paws by slowly increasing the duration of your walks.

Before making your dog your exercise buddy, the first step is a veterinary checkup. Your vet will check your dog's heart, lungs, and overall health to ensure they're fit for fitness. As our dogs age, a joint and mobility check is recommended. Dogs with joint or ligament inflammation may need a low-impact exercise plan, such as swimming or walking.

SAMPLE WORKOUTS

Continue to challenge yourself with a daily routine that includes a brisk, warm-up walk followed by jogging or running intervals. Slow down and rest as needed. Incorporate play like fetch or agility training, and finish with a cooldown walk. Check the weather and adjust on hot, sweltering days. Exercise in the morning when it's cooler. Always bring water for you and your dog and monitor both your energy levels.

EDUCATIONAL INSIGHTS

- Consult Your Veterinarian: Always check with your vet before starting a new exercise routine with your dog.
- Know Your Dog's Limits: Be aware of breed-specific needs and limitations.
- Hydrate Frequently and Take Breaks: Especially in hot weather.

- Protect Their Paws: Use protective gear like booties to safeguard your dog's paws from harsh surfaces.
- Increase Activity Gradually: Prevent overexertion by increasing the intensity and duration over time.

STORY

Once an energetic soul with a vigor for life, 68-year-old Sally found herself confined to her home as age and a hip injury caught up with her. Her once-brisk walks with her faithful companion, Buddy, had become a distant memory. Each step was a challenge; her joints ached with every step, and her energy dwindled. But Sally wasn't one to surrender easily. Determined to reclaim her former vitality, she began a gradual rehabilitation journey, with Buddy faithfully by her side. It began with short, hesitant steps in the hallway, as she used her walker for support. Buddy nudged her gently forward, his eyes filled with encouragement as if urging her to keep going with each step. The thoughts of her physical therapist echoed, "You've got this!" in her mind as she built up enough strength to transition to her cane.

With each passing day, Sally pushed herself a little further. On perfect Minnesota summer days, she ventured into the garden, leaning on her cane for support, while Buddy trotted beside her, his tail wagging in approval. The fresh air and warm sunlight breathed new life into her weary bones, and Sally felt hope ignite within her with each step.

Despite the setbacks and moments of frustration (which are normal during any recovery), Sally persevered. She joined gentle exercise classes for seniors, where she met others on the same journey toward mobility and independence. Together, they cheered each other on, celebrating even the smallest victories, sharing stories about their dogs.

As the weeks turned into months, Sally's progress was remarkable. Her steps grew steadier and more balanced. Her confidence soared with each successful outing. Buddy, her ever-faithful companion, remained her constant source of inspiration, his unwavering loyalty a testament to their enduring bond.

One perfect afternoon, Sally made a decision. Dressed in her walking shoes and holding Buddy's leash, she stepped outside with a newfound determination and a glimpse of her former self returning. The pavement stretched before her, urging her forward. She knew this was the moment she had worked so hard for—physical therapy, her exercise classes, and now the light shining on her to bring it all together. With an ear-to-ear smile and a sparkle in her eyes, Sally took her first step without her cane. Her gait was slow and cautious at first, but she gradually gained momentum and control. Beside her, Buddy walked proudly, his tail wagging in rhythm with her steps, as if to say, "We're doing it, Ma! We're doing it together!"

Sally reclaimed a part of herself with each step—the spirited, adventurous woman she had always been. Walking beside Buddy, she discovered that age was just a number and that the path to vitality was best traveled with a faithful friend by her side. She regained her independence, taking the time to live fully, slowly, and safely again.

Everyone gets the chance to be young, but not everyone gets a chance to be old.
—Jennifer Erdmann, a physical therapist and spine specialist
Embrace life.

RECOMMENDATIONS

- Check with Your Veterinarian: Consult them before starting a new exercise routine for your dog.
- Set a Weekly Goal: Aim for at least 150 minutes of moderate-intensity exercise a week for yourself.
- Increase Gradually: Prevent injuries by slowly building up intensity and duration over time.
- Stay Hydrated: Always bring enough water for you and your dog, especially in warm weather.
- Protect Their Paws: Use protective gear like dog booties to shield your dog's paws from harmful surfaces.
- Adapt to the Weather: Adjust exercise plans accordingly.
- Choose Joint-Friendly Activities: Incorporate low-impact exercises like swimming for older dogs and those with joint issues.

SUMMARY

Confront challenges as they arise and take proactive steps to ensure your and your dog's safety and well-being. Teaching your dog commands like *heel* can be a lifesaver. Maintaining a regular exercise routine can prevent injuries and promote longevity. Remember, your proactive steps today can save you from reactive struggles tomorrow.

CHAPTER 18

TROTTING AND WAGGING: FETCHING IS FUN!

Injury prevention and brain health are crucial components of maintaining both your own health and your dog's health. Moving and engaging in exercise are some of the best ways to prevent injuries by strengthening muscles, improving coordination, and building mental resilience. By incorporating these practices into your daily routine, you can enjoy the benefits of a healthier lifestyle while also strengthening your bond with your dog.

HUMAN ELEMENT

Before we dive into what *fetch* means, let's recap what we've learned so far:

- Strategies to overcome barriers to exercise
- How to build a supportive team and seek guidance
- Developed actionable plans
- Chewed on ways to support our pack
- How to match our activity levels with those of our dogs
- Resets are essential in life
- How our ages can guide us
- The fuselage and why it compares to our core

- Adventures throughout our lives are a necessary ingredient
- We've journeyed through time, exploring how to stay passionate at every stage of life
- How adaptation requires time
- We've marveled at the amazing human body
- We have learned that the most important thing is to keep moving and establish a battle rhythm

Occasionally, we must *heel*. What's next, you say? Fetch!

Walking is a simple, cost-effective way to stay active that can be easily integrated into your daily routine. Setting time, distance, or fun terrain goals can make walking more enjoyable and challenging. Jogging or running are other excellent options, but remember to listen to your body and gradually build intensity to prevent overuse injuries.

Strength training exercises, such as resistance bands or bodyweight movements, help build muscle and prevent injuries. Incorporating activities that enhance balance and coordination like yoga or tai chi can also reduce the risk of falls and improve overall stability. By following these guidelines and engaging in activities you enjoy, you can maintain a healthy and active lifestyle, reducing the likelihood of injuries and improving your overall well-being.

Ensure you're fully present when you're with your dog. Eliminate distractions; life is busy, but your time with your dog is limited. Sadly, throughout our lives, we'll experience the loss of our dogs due to their shorter life expectancy. I strongly encourage you to be present and intentional with your precious time. Enjoy these moments, every single day. By being present and intentional, you will value and cherish these memories for a lifetime.

Let the activities and creativity flow as you play fetch with your dog. Your only limitation is your imagination. Be innovative. Most importantly, move. I'm going to start with the basics and then toss out some other unique ideas. As I say to my patients, "You must master the basics and earn the right to progress. Remember, your fuselage must be strong enough to support your arms and legs."

It's time to pause and reflect. Use the following as a stepping stone to movement and other activities:

- Lead the Pack: Take charge and have fun each week
- Laugh Daily: A little humor makes it fun
- Be Creative: Dream big and innovate
- Stay Present: In every moment of movement, be engaged
- Value Each Moment: Appreciate the time you have with your dog
- No Regrets: Focus on creating positive memories

Be the pack leader and have fun throughout each week. A daily dose of laughter will make it fun. Be creative, dream, and innovate; in that moment of movement, be present. Appreciate and value each moment. Don't have regrets, just positive memories. Remember, you don't *have* to do these activities—you *get* to. Consider them blessings rather than tasks.

DOG CARE

Fetching with our dogs is simple. Toss a ball or other object and then wait for them to return it. If you peel back a few more layers, *fetch* reveals much more. It's the act of being intentional and present. Eyes locked, breathing steady, muscles tense, and the release of the object causes excitement, purpose, and joy. The sprint. The wagging tail. Your dog returns the object, pleased with the effort, and sits grounded, balanced, and ready to repeat, again and again. Playing fetch is a classic activity that provides physical exercise and stimulates your dog's mental acuity.

Matching the activity to your dog's needs and capabilities is important. Watch for signs of fatigue or discomfort and adjust the intensity and duration as needed.

Agility training is another fun way to keep your dog active; it improves their coordination, balance, and overall fitness. This can include setting up obstacle courses with tunnels, jumps, and weave poles.

SAMPLE WORKOUTS

Warm-Up (5-10 minutes):

- Walk: Begin with a brisk walk on a new path, trail, or hill to warm up both you and your dog.
- Stretch: Gently perform dynamic stretches while also loosening up your dog's legs to prepare for the workout.

Main Workout (20-30 minutes):

- Fetch: Throw a ball or flying disk for your dog to fetch. While your dog is running, perform bodyweight exercises like squats, lunges, or push-ups.

- Jogging: Run around the park or neighborhood, allowing your dog to keep pace with you.
- Agility Training: Set up cones, tunnels, and jumps. Guide your dog through the course while performing similar movements yourself.

Cool Down (5-10 minutes):

- Walk: Slow down the pace with a gentle walk to bring your heart rate back to normal.
- Stretch: Finish with a series of deep stretches for both you and your dog to prevent stiffness and promote flexibility.

EDUCATIONAL INSIGHTS

- Dog Motivation: Dogs move and fetch because it's done with a purpose. Make sure to provide a rewarding purpose that keeps that tail wagging!
- Human Motivation: Intrinsic motivation and drive need to be guided by happiness and movement.
- Mental Focus: Incorporate intentional rest, puzzles, toys, and training exercises to keep your dog's mind sharp and engaged.

STORY

One sunny afternoon, I sat at home with my little brother and older sister, watching our dog, Sir Ruffagus, play in the yard. I bet my little brother that he couldn't beat my older sister in a game of fetch. "It's on," he said. I tossed the ball as far as possible, and my brother sprinted after it with all his might. Just as he was halfway, my sister, who had remained motionless, said, "Fetch." Sir Ruffagus, understanding the command, darted past my brother, grabbed the ball, and returned it to my sister, who smiled victoriously. It was a simple game, but it reminded us of the joy of being present and cherishing these moments with our beloved pets.

Imagine you've had a long, stressful day at work. You come home feeling drained and overwhelmed. Sensing your mood, your dog eagerly greets you at the door with his wagging tail. You decide to take a walk together, enjoying the fresh air and the simple pleasure of your dog's company. As you walk, the stress begins to melt away, replaced by a sense of calmness and connection. This simple act of walking your dog improves your physical health and provides emotional relief, illustrating the profound impact our furry friends can have on our lives.

RECOMMENDATIONS

- Schedule Regular Walks: Set a daily schedule for walks with your dog to ensure consistent exercise.
- Incorporate Variety: Mix up activities like jogging, fetch, swimming, and agility training to keep both you and your dog engaged and challenged.
- Monitor Health: Regularly check both your and your dog's health, looking for signs of fatigue, discomfort, or potential injuries.

- Be Present: Focus on being present and enjoying the time spent with your dog, creating lasting memories.

SUMMARY

The best way to predict your future is to create it.
—Peter Drucker

Integrating regular exercise and injury prevention practices into your routine can create a healthier, happier future for you and your dog. Move better together! Whether it's a simple walk or a playful game of fetch, these activities improve physical health and deepen the bond between you and your furry friend. Keep moving, stay present, and cherish every moment spent together.

Now, what's next? Fetch!

CHAPTER 19

WALKING AND OTHER ADVENTURES

Walking is one of the most natural and cost-effective forms of movement. Not only is it free, but it's also a fantastic way to prevent injury, build endurance, and maintain good health. The bonus? Your dog loves it just as much as you do! Walking is the perfect activity to keep both you and your furry friend fit, without requiring expensive equipment or gym memberships.

HUMAN ELEMENT

Walking can be transformed into a fun and customizable exercise. You can set goals for distance, speed, or terrain. Whether you're walking briskly for a cardiovascular workout, enjoying a leisurely stroll, or even mixing things up with sideways and backward steps, the key is to keep moving. Walking naturally transitions into jogging or running, which adds intensity to your workouts. With proper progression, it also keeps you balanced and injury-free. For those seeking variety, the options are endless—from exploring new trails to joining a local walking group or enjoying urban adventures.

For those who love water-based activities, swimming is an excellent low-impact workout. It strengthens cardiovascular fitness, improves mobility, and works nearly all your muscles; it's also gentle on your joints. Whether it's land- or water-based activities, the goal is to stay moving, prevent injury, and enjoy the process.

DOG CARE

Your dog is your best exercise companion, whether you're walking, jogging, or even swimming. Not all dogs are built for running, but with the right approach, your furry friend can be an eager participant in your fitness routine. For instance, my shih tzu, Einstein, could jog three miles! Larger dogs, like my vizsla, Edison, can easily handle much longer distances.

Pay attention to your dog's needs; if they're panting heavily or lagging, it's time for a break. Dogs don't sweat like humans and rely on panting to cool down, so watch the temperature and time of day when exercising. Adventure-seekers can also explore canicross, an activity where dogs are harnessed to their humans for running or even swimming together. Whatever the activity, the joy of exercising with your dog is undeniable.

SAMPLE WORKOUTS

- Start with a 30-minute walk: Gradually increase the speed.
- Warm-up: For 10 minutes, incorporate 5 minutes of brisk walking, 5 minutes of side shuffling, and a 2-minute break, or power walk as fast as you can for your chosen duration.
- Catch! For an added challenge, bring a ball to toss to your dog during breaks.

- Cooldown: Wind down with light stretches and a leisurely stroll home.

EDUCATIONAL INSIGHTS

Here are some reminders:

- Keep water and snacks handy during long walks or hikes.
- Dogs can develop fitness like humans—start slowly and build up.
- Use the 10 percent rule by increasing your dog's activity by no more than 10 percent a week to prevent injury.

STORY

One of my proudest moments was when Einstein, my shih tzu, accompanied me on a three-mile jog. She was a little tank and kept pace like a pro! The funny part was that most people couldn't believe a small dog like her could go that distance. She showed that even the smallest dogs can tackle the big challenges with the right training.

Imagine it's a sunny day, and you've decided to take your dog for a jog. You're feeling energized, but halfway through, your dog starts slowing down. You check the temperature—too hot for such intense activity. You stop, offer water, and decide to switch to a shaded trail at a slower pace. Your dog's tail wags in appreciation, and you both finish the jog feeling refreshed. This moment of empathy and adaptability highlights the importance of listening to your body—and your dog's—during exercise.

RECOMMENDATIONS

- Set a walking or jogging goal for you and your dog for the week (e.g., 20 minutes, three times a week).
- Keep water and a collapsible water bowl handy during activities.
- Observe your dog's energy levels during walks and adjust the exercise intensity accordingly.
- Explore new terrains or activities like swimming or hiking to challenge both of you.
- Make sure you're both stretching and cooling down after each workout.
- Create your "Paw"pared Packing List, (a.k.a. Your Dog's Go Bag Checklist in Appendix B).

SUMMARY

Movement is life—whether it's you or your dog, keeping active is key to a happier, healthier lifestyle. So lace up, leash up, and get moving, my move-better-together adventurers!

TIP #20
INNOVATE.
BE INTENTIONAL AND PRESENT.

CHAPTER 20

THINGS TO DO AND OTHER FUN ACTIVITIES

Here's a "paw-some" encore of fun and creative ways to make lasting memories together:

- Walking:
    - Set goals for time, distance, terrain, or elevation.
    - Try walking briskly, sideways, backward, or even freestyle.
- Jogging/Running:
    - Gradually build up your dog's endurance.
    - Use the 10 percent rule to avoid overuse injuries.
- Canicross (Dog-Powered Running): Use a bungee harness when running with dogs.
- Swimming:
    - A great low-impact exercise for you and your dog.
    - Use treats or toys to encourage dogs that are new to water.
- Doggy Paddle and Water Fetch: Play fetch in the water to burn energy and keep cool.
- Kayaking or Canoeing: A core workout for you and a balance exercise for your dog.
- Hiking: Explore trails to experience fresh air and varied terrain.

- Fetch and Fit: Combine fetch with bodyweight exercises, such as squats, lunges, push-ups, and planks.
- High-Intensity Interval Training (HIIT) Fetch: Sprint after the ball while playing fetch to raise your heart rate.
- Dog Park: This is a great opportunity for your dog to explore off-leash and socialize while you walk around.
- Agility Courses: Jog and guide your dog through obstacles like tunnels and jumps.
- Hunting: Engage your dog in retrieving or flushing games for hunting breeds.
- Soccer: Play gentle games of keep-away or work on footwork with a soccer ball.
- Tug-of-War: Engage in gentle tugging games, but be mindful of your dog's teeth and spine.
- Biking /Rollerblading: Ride alongside your dog or use a bike trailer for smaller or less active dogs.
- Dog Scootering: Let your dog pull you on a non-motorized scooter for fun and exercise.
- Skijoring (winter activity): Cross-country skiing with your dog harnessed to you for snow-filled fun.
- Snowshoeing: Trek through the snow while canicrossing with your dog.
- Wrestling: Engage in playful and controlled wrestling on the floor.
- Dancing with Your Dog: Dance to your favorite music with your dog as your partner.
- Trick Training: Teach tricks like sit, stay, roll over, high-five, army crawl or even advanced tricks like grabbing a beverage.

- Hide-and-Seek: Hide treats or toys for your dog to sniff out and find.
- LARPing (Live Action Role-Playing): Dress up and role-play with your dog in a fantasy or historical setting.
- Snoozing/Resting: Don't forget to recharge with quality rest after a full day of activity.
- Obstacle Course
    - Set up a simple obstacle course in your yard or home using household items like chairs, cones, or broomsticks.
    - Have your dog navigate through tunnels, jump over objects, and weave through obstacles.
- Scent Work: Hide scented objects or treats around your home or yard for your dog to find. This stimulates their minds and uses their natural scenting abilities. Scent work is mentally enriching and physically engaging.
- Flying Disk (Disk Dog): Perfect for fetching, improving agility, and enhancing your dog's cardiovascular fitness. Some dogs can catch disks in midair!
- Treadmill Training:
    - When outdoor activity isn't an option, try training your dog to walk or jog on a treadmill.
    - Start slowly and always supervise to ensure safety.
- Dog Yoga (Doga): Incorporate yoga with your dog. This combines gentle movements, stretches, and bonding time with your dog while enhancing your flexibility.
- Hide-and-Seek with Family Members: Have a family member hide in the house or yard while your dog tries to find them. It's a great mental challenge and fun for everyone involved.
- Paddleboarding:

- If you're near a lake or calm body of water, stand-up paddleboarding can be a fun way for both you and your dog to exercise.
- Ensure your dog is comfortable in the water and consider using life vests.
- Dog-Friendly Group Fitness Classes:
  - Some fitness classes are specifically designed for owners and their dogs, incorporating strength training, stretching, and cardiovascular activities.
  - Look for local options like Bark Bootcamp, Doga, or similar offerings.
- Canine Freestyle (Dog Dancing): Take dancing with your dog to the next level by learning choreographed routines to music. This can be a fun and engaging way to bond while improving coordination and training.
- Couch-to-5K Dog Training: Many 5-kilometer events now feature dog-friendly races, allowing you and your furry partner to train together toward a common goal.
- Tracking or Trail Running: Train your dog in tracking skills on a nature trail or open field. This engages their natural hunting instincts, increasing mental stimulation during walks and runs.
- Camping and Backpacking:
  - Take your dog on a camping trip where they can experience new surroundings, scents, and adventures.
  - For backpacking, consider having your dog carry their gear in a pack as part of their exercise routine.
- Dog-Friendly Fitness Apps: These can guide you through exercises that incorporate your dog in activities such as running, bodyweight exercises, or mobility workouts.

- Canoeing/Boating:
    - Consider a relaxed day of canoeing or boating with your dog
    - Make sure your dog is comfortable around water and wears a canine life jacket
- Dog Soccer (Jolly Ball): Some dogs love playing with large balls. Organize a fun game where your dog can chase and kick the ball around the yard, providing lots of fun and exercise.

The true sign of intelligence is not knowledge but imagination.
—Albert Einstein

CONCLUSION

Sniff, sniff. Waggle, Waggle. My animal instincts are sensing your urgency to incorporate Dog'ercise into your routine for a happier, more active life with your dog. The 21 Tips throughout this book will help you and your dog stay healthy and injury-free.

The goal is simple: Just keep moving. Stay accountable for maintaining movement and inertia for both you and your dog. Both you and your dog, now and in the future, will enjoy life as you stay motivated to keep moving. While it's easy to get overwhelmed by too much information, don't let analysis lead to paralysis. Focus on you, the athlete, and keep moving alongside your dog. Move better together!

Keep moving and make your dog part of your fitness routine. As the saying goes, *Health is wealth*. Staying active together leads to a healthier, happier, and more fulfilling life for both you and your dog. Remember, it's not about perfection but steady progress and enjoying the journey together.

Walking and spending time with your dog is always worthwhile. It helps maintain your inertia and creates companionship with your dog and family. Don't let the fear of injury stop you from being active. Keep moving! The risks associated with a sedentary lifestyle are far greater than the risks of movement.

Just move. And what better way to do it than with your best friend, your dog? How you move doesn't matter—just move, be safe, and live for adventure. Lead by example for your pack and create a legacy for future generations. By doing so, we'll make the world a better place, one paw and foot at a time. That's the ultimate dog rule—live for adventure, cherish the companionship, and move better together. You've got this! *Ruff! Ruff!*

TIP #21

MAINTAIN COMPANIONSHIP. SEEK ADVENTURES.

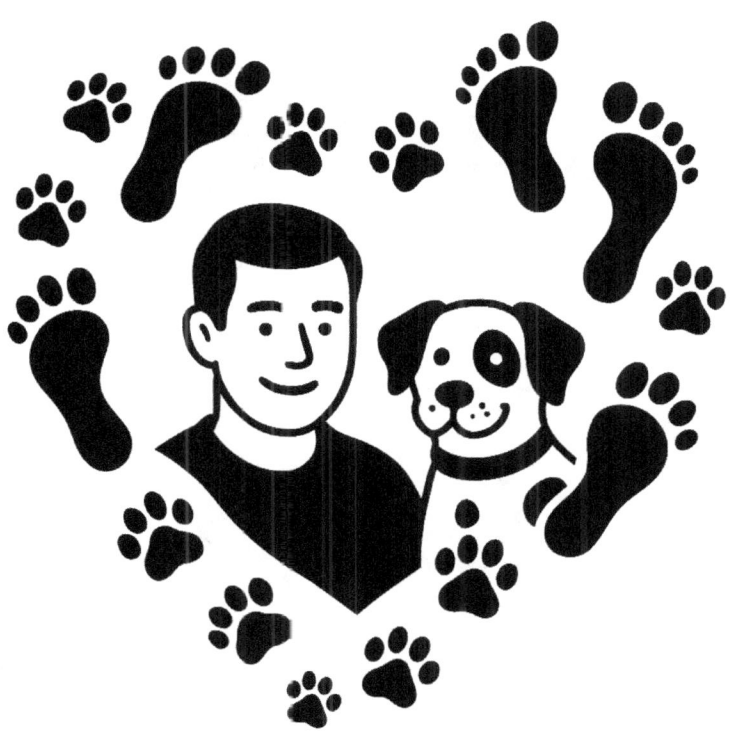

Thanks for reading this book! I hope you've found it useful, educational, and a lot of fun.

21 TIPS FOR A HEALTHY, INJURY-FREE LIFE

For more healthy tips on exercising with your dog, sign up for my newsletter at www.movebettertogether.com.

Your journey doesn't end here. Scan to move better, live well, and connect.

Move Better Together website

Brandon Schomberg's website

ACKNOWLEDGMENTS

To my incredible family, the stars of my life's sitcom: To my beautiful wife, the queen of my heart and the CEO of our topsy-turvy but love-filled household. Your ability to turn chaos into harmony is truly magical. To my amazing kids, who somehow manage to be both the reasons I lose my mind and can't stop smiling. Your energy and laughter are the secret ingredients to our daily chaos stew, and our two four-legged companions, the canine maestros of mayhem—the *real* bosses of the house—our dogs, living proof that unconditional love and muddy paw prints go hand in paw. And to those who doubt my ability to inspire greatness, look how I convinced the kids to eat broccoli (sometimes) or how the dogs "willingly" go on diets. If that's not persuasive prowess, I don't know what it is.

Amid this organized frenzy, a serious mission is at play. My dedication to promoting healthier lives is fueled by the desire for humans and dogs to lead long, joyful lives, much like the daily parade of squeaky toys in our living room.

In our household, we don't just dream big—we dream dog-sized dreams and chase them with the enthusiasm of a kid in a candy store. So, here's to living our best lives, embracing mayhem, and inspiring everyone (humans and dogs alike) to reach their full potential. With love, laughter, and a trail of dog treats, please follow along as we "live for adventure and stay happy by moving better together."

Brandon Schomberg

APPENDIX A

THE DOG LEASH GUIDE

Dog leashes come in various types and styles, each designed for specific activities, dog sizes, ages, environments, and training levels.

Choose leashes based on your dog's age, activity level, and environment. Consider factors such as size, strength, and your surroundings. Use shorter leashes for puppies or urban areas and longer ones for open spaces. Having the right leash ensures you're prepared for any setting, so you can remain active, have fun, and keep your dog safe.

- Standard Leashes: Ideal for daily walks and basic training sessions. They are typically 4–8 feet long, made of nylon or leather, and are suitable for all ages and sizes. Puppies benefit from using smaller leashes, while larger breeds require stronger, reinforced options that are resistant to wear.
- No-Pull Harness Leashes: This style distributes pressure along the body, reducing pulling and providing better control across the chest.
- Chain Leashes: These are suitable for dogs that pull strongly but may be too cumbersome and heavy for smaller dogs.

- Long Leashes: These range from 8 to over 100 feet. They are perfect for recall training or exploration and are best used with harnesses for safety. Great for roaming in open spaces.
- Traffic Leads: These are short (18 inches long) and designed for close control in crowded areas. Ideal for large or energetic dogs in busy urban environments, providing better control in crowded spaces.
- Bungee Leashes: These elastic, shock-absorbing leashes are often hands-free and are ideal for running or hiking. They are not suitable for dogs that pull strongly.
- Retractable Leashes Allow for variable lengths but require caution to avoid tangling or accidents. Best suited for smaller, well-trained dogs, but are not recommended for larger breeds due to a lack of control and a higher risk of pulling.
- Slip Leads: Ideal for strong pullers as they will tighten gently when the dog pulls, helping to discourage pulling behavior.

APPENDIX B

THE "PAW"PARED PACKING LIST

(a.k.a. Your Dog's Go Bag Checklist)

Available at www.movebettertogether.com as a free downloadable PDF.

Packing these essentials ensures you and your dog stay safe, hydrated, and ready for whatever adventure lies ahead!

Must-Have Items:

- Leash: For safety and control during walks or hikes.
- Collapsible Water Bowl: Portable and easy to use, keeping your dog hydrated.
- Water Jug: Bring enough water for both you and your dog, especially on longer adventures and warmer days.
- Towel: Great for cleaning off after a swim or muddy outing.
- Doggy Bags: Always be prepared for cleanup.
- Snacks/Food: Pack energy-boosting snacks for you and your dog.
- Fully Charged Phone (or a portable charger): Keep it handy for emergencies or navigation.
- Sunscreen and Lip Balm: Protect yourself from the sun's harmful rays.

- Flashlight: If you're out longer than planned.
- Dog ID and Medical Records: Ensure your dog has proper identification and bring any necessary health information.
- Medications: If you or your dog requires any medications, remember to bring them.
- Reflective Gear: Provides visibility during early morning or evening outings.
- Emergency Contact List: A list of important phone numbers and contacts to use in the event of an emergency.
- Money: Bring cash, a credit card, or set up bank info on your phone.

Exercise Gear:
- Resistance Bands: Lightweight and versatile for a quick workout on the go.
- Flying Disk or Ball: Perfect for a game of fetch to keep your dog engaged and active.
- Jump Rope: A quick cardiovascular boost if you want to squeeze in some extra movement.
- Foam Roller: Post-exercise recovery to help relax tight muscles.

Optional but Highly Recommended:
- First Aid Kit: To handle minor injuries for humans and dogs.
- Wet/Cold/Hot Weather Gear: Be prepared for changing conditions.
- Map: Especially if you're heading into unfamiliar territory.
- Extra Shoes and Socks: In case you encounter wet or muddy conditions.
- Multi-Tool or Knife: Handy for various outdoor situations.

- Blanket: Useful for resting spots or chilly weather.
- Solar Charger: To keep your devices charged if you're out for an extended time.

APPENDIX C

RECOMMENDED WEBSITES

How do you choose the *right* dog?

When considering adopting a dog, it's essential to thoroughly understand the responsibilities involved. Many trustworthy websites offer valuable information to help families choose the ideal canine companion, and it's just a few clicks away.

When selecting a dog for your family, gather information from multiple sources and consider factors such as size, energy level, grooming requirements, and temperament. Always conduct thorough research and if possible, consider adopting from reputable shelters or rescue organizations. Breed-specific rescue organizations or clubs can offer helpful guidance in finding the perfect furry companion for your family.

Here is a selected list of resources to help you make well-informed decisions. The website links are provided for educational purposes only. The author is not responsible for any information or points of view on these sites.

American Kennel Club (AKC)
- Website: https://www.akc.org/
- Provides resources and guides to help families find a suitable dog breed that matches their lifestyle, preferences, and needs.

- Information about various breeds, their characteristics, and important factors to consider when selecting a dog is available.
- Offers resources on responsible dog ownership, training, and health.

Local Animal Humane Society: Find your local animal humane society
- Website: https://bestfriends.org/pet-care-resources/bringing-new-dog-home-what-know
- Website: https://www.carverscotths.org/adopterswelcome Many dogs are available for adoption, and the local staff can help you find the perfect match for your family with their knowledge and guidance.

Humane World for Animals: Adopting a Dog Guide
- Website: https://www.humaneworld.org/en/resources/how-bring-your-new-dog-home-and-make-them-feel-welcome
- This guide offers valuable insights on how to adopt a dog responsibly. It discusses factors to consider when selecting the right pet for your family, emphasizing the importance of responsible ownership.

Petfinder
- Website: https://www.petfinder.com/
- Petfinder is a platform that connects potential adopters with pets available for adoption
- Highlights the importance of responsible adoption and offers a wide range of dogs from shelters and rescue organizations.
- Provides information about various breeds.

ASPCA Adopt a Pet
- Website: https://www.aspca.org/adopt-pet
- Provides guidance on adopting pets, including tips for selecting the right one for your family. Their resources address various aspects of responsible pet ownership.

Dog Time
- Website: https://dogtime.com/
- Offers a wealth of resources on various dog breeds and information on training and care.
- Breed selector tool helps families find suitable breeds based on their preferences, ensuring a more informed decision-making process.

The Spruce Pets: Choosing the Right Dog for Your Family
- Website: https://www.thesprucepets.com/dog-breeds-4162141
- Offers articles and guides on various aspects of pet ownership, including how to select the right dog for your family.
- The content provides key factors to consider and provides helpful tips for responsible adoption.

International Association of Canine Professionals (IACP)
- Website: https://iacpdogs.org/
- Leading professional association of dog trainers, behavior consultants, and canine professionals around the globe.
- Focuses on professional dog training and behavior, but has many resources that can be valuable for dog owners seeking to learn about training progressions and milestones.

Association of Professional Dog Trainers (APDT)
- Website: https://apdt.com/
- Promotes positive dog-training methods and offers several resources and articles to help dog owners.
- Includes a directory of certified professional dog trainers to help with training or behavioral problems.

The American Veterinary Society of Animal Behavior (AVSAB)
- Website: https://avsab.org/
- Veterinarians and professionals dedicated to the understanding and promotion of animal behavior.
- Provides information on behavioral milestones and contributes to overall animal well-being.

Pet Professional Guild (PPG)
- Website: https://www.petprofessionalguild.com/
- Focuses on force-free pet care and training.
- Provides resources for dog owners on positive reinforcement training and behavior modification.

UK Kennel Club (KC)
- Website: https://www.thekennelclub.org.uk/
- Based in the United Kingdom, one of the oldest and most influential kennel clubs globally.
- Registers purebred dogs, organizes dog shows, and promotes responsible dog ownership.
- Provides information on various breeds, health screening programs, and resources for dog owners.

Continental Kennel Club
- Website: https://ckcusa.com/
- An all-breed canine registry that publishes breed standards and details.
- Resource for dog breeders and owners, providing education and support for registration solutions and certifications.

Fédération Cynologique Internationale (FCI)
- Website: https://www.fci.be/en/
- Serves as the international umbrella organization for national kennel clubs worldwide
- Establishes breed standards, organizes international dog shows, and promotes cooperation among its member organizations.

ABOUT THE AUTHOR

Brandon Schomberg is a board-certified doctor of physical therapy, an American soldier, and an enthusiastic advocate for healthy, active living for both people and their dogs. He lives in Minnesota with his wife, three children, and two dogs. Drawing on years of clinical experience and military leadership, Brandon leads a multidisciplinary team at Twin Cities Orthopedics. He serves as the director of the Sports Physical Therapy Residency program while also developing specialty programs across TCO. Outside work, he stays active with his family, walking the dogs, and hitting the golf course, where movement and mindfulness meet. Brandon is equally passionate about leadership, personal growth, and lifelong learning—often found with a book that helps him grow as a clinician, mentor, and person. In his book *Healthy Living with Your Dog: 21 Tips for a Healthy Injury-Free Life*, he introduces "Dog'ercise," a fun and functional approach to bonding with your dog while building a more active lifestyle. With practical tools, military-inspired motivation, and humor, Brandon encourages readers to "Charlie Mike"—continue the mission—and move better together.

Move Better Together website

Brandon Schomberg's website

www.ingramcontent.com/pod-product-compliance
Lightning Source LLC
Chambersburg PA
CBHW070622030426
42337CB00020B/3883